EXPLORATIONS IN AUTISM

EXPLORATIONS IN AUTISM
A PSYCHOANALYTICAL STUDY

Donald Meltzer

with

John Bremner
Shirley Hoxter
Doreen Weddell
Isca Wittenberg

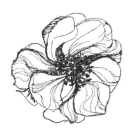

THE HARRIS MELTZER TRUST

First published in 1975 by Clunie Press for The Roland Harris Educational Trust
Republished in 2008 by Karnac Books for The Harris Meltzer Trust
New edition 2018 by The Harris Meltzer Trust
60 New Caledonian Wharf
London SE16 7TW

British Library Cataloguing in Publication Data
A C.I.P. for this book is available from the British Library

ISBN 978 1 912567 48 5

Edited, designed and produced by The Bourne Studios
www.bournestudios.co.uk
Printed in Great Britain
www.harris-meltzer-trust.org.uk

CONTENTS

FOREWORD *by Meg Harris Williams*   vii

SECTION A: THEORY

1 Aims, scope and method of the investigation
   Donald Meltzer   1

2 The psychology of autistic states and of post-autistic
   mentality
   Donald Meltzer   5

SECTION B: CLINICAL FINDINGS

INTRODUCTION by Donald Meltzer   33

3 Autism proper: Timmy
   John Bremner   35

4 Primal depression in autism: John
   Isca Wittenberg   57

5 Disturbed geography of the life-space in autism: Barry
   Doreen Weddell   99

6 The residual autistic condition and its effect upon
      learning: Piffie
      Shirley Hoxter   159

7 Mutism in autism, schizophrenia and manic-depressive
      states - the correlation of clinical psychopathology
      and linguistics
      Donald Meltzer   191

SECTION C: IMPLICATIONS

8 The relation of autism to obsessional states in general
      Donald Meltzer   209

9 Dimensionality in mental functioning
      Donald Meltzer   225

10 Conclusion
       Donald Meltzer   241

BIBLIOGRAPHY   247

CHRONOLOGY OF TREATMENT PROCESSES   249

AUTHOR AND SUBJECT INDEX   255

ACKNOWLEDGEMENTS

The preliminary studies leading to the writing of this book were generously supported by the Melanie Klein Trust.

We are indebted to Meg Harris for copying the drawings of Chapter 5.

The authors have contributed their sections so that this book could be published by, and for the benefit of, The Roland Harris Educational Trust.

T his book, founded on investigations by a group of child analysts supervised by Donald Meltzer in the mid 1960s to early 70s, is a pioneering work in many ways: first and foremost in its clinical description of the nature of childhood autism (then little understood), but also in the fundamental shift posited in the psychoanalytic view of the mind in general, particularly with reference to aesthetic experience and the development of language. The struggle to understand the emotional impact of the children's transference enabled a special use of the new ideas of Esther Bick and Wilfred Bion about dimensionality and mindlessness which amplified Melanie Klein's vision of the psychic reality of the inner world and its objects. Meltzer did say later that in subsequent years the definition of autism became widened and perhaps also diluted, but that the original picture of autistic and post-autistic states in specific children who are acutely sensitive to sensory bombardment, made it possible to generalise about potentially ubiquitous mental processes of dismantling and two-dimensionality, in the sense of being part of everyone's mental equipment (or its disabling).

Meltzer's own countertransference to the group of children documented in this book, he says, was to a 'compound individual' at different stages of an autistic illness; and this is how the clinical cases are presented and indexed, to illustrate the economics and dynamics of the autistic state as exemplified by children of very different personalities. These findings are then extended to clinical work with adults, in the service of exploring problems of language and communication: the mutism or speech deficiencies that are intrinsic to autism – owing to the incapacity to internalise a 'speaking object' with whom they desire to communicate – have parallel manifestations in adults, as does the expanded insight into special types of obsessionality, as distinct from ordinary narcissism.

Meltzer disliked the quest for causes of psychopathology (which he considered a quasi-scientific illusion) but he points out that the focus on the cases of these children suggests that autism is more constitutional than environmental, and pertains to characters who are innately vulnerable to catastrophic depressive experience, adhesively possessive of their object to the extent that no separation (hence sense of time or space) is tolerable, hence no internalisation; who are by nature non-sadistic so instead of achieving splitting-and-idealization they turn to dismantling of their own mental structures, something that is experienced in the countertransference as the equivalent of a petit-mal attack on communication, a suspension of mental life, rather than of a move to a different level of transference communication. It is also, suggests Meltzer, at the root of substituting 'transitional objects' for real ones. Such children, or child-parts of the self, avoid anxiety and despair by allowing themselves to temporarily fall apart whilst remaining adhesively identified with their object in a non-conflictual arrangement. This involves an unusual degree of dependence on the functions as well as the services of the object, something which may in fact compound the problems faced by the mother figure, exacerbating the situation. These children, in their non-trustful obsessionality, have a sense of permeability, and of the permeability of their object. Essentially they have difficulty in building an internal world of phantasy in Meltzer's sense of a 'theatre for the generation of meaning'. Hence the frequent impression of premature oldness, of having achieved a Wordsworthian recollection-in-tranquillity at a time of life that should be ruled by emotional turbulence, and when there has not been enough experience to recollect, tranquilly or otherwise.

Yet the reader, affected by the vividness of the analysts' depictions of their experience, will also empathise with the 'heroic' impression made on Meltzer by these children who refuse to fight and activate whatever 'germ of greatness' lies within them, through a potential Kierkegaardian leap in the dark; and with their ingenious methods of avoiding immersion in the conflictual human condition. They have not yet realised that there is no solution other than to develop ego-strength, something which according to Meltzer has only become comprehensible in psychoanalytic terms since the advent of Bion's concept of container–contained and Bick's of the skin-container function (although he differentiates autism's 'spacelessness' from 'second-skin').

I would like to reinforce this brief and informal preface (by a non-practitioner) with quotations from reviews by some of the clinicians outside this book who worked with Meltzer in the course of treating autistic or post-autistic children. Carmo di Sousa Lima (of the Portuguese Psychoanalytical Society) writes about dimensionality and the dynamics of the transference:

> *Explorations in Autism* is a turning-point in both the understanding of and the clinical approach to autism. The clinical material gradually unveils the geography of the internal mother (which proved crucial for the development of Meltzer's 'claustrum' theory) and allowed him to draft, for the first time in psychoanalysis, a theory of the dimensionality of mental life. The book, furthermore, is a moving journey through the dynamics of the transference–countertransference, revealing what Meltzer calls 'the essentials of humanity'. It should be part of the training of every analyst and I believe it would be a revelation to many philosophers of the mind.

Didier Houzel (of the French Psychoanalytical Association) writes of the expanded model of the mind:

> The rigorous exploration reported in this book has shed a totally new light on the subjective experience of autistic children and hence on the primitive developmental phases of every human mind. A new metapsychological model of the psyche stems from the description here of fundamental

concepts like primal depression, dismantling, adhesive identity, dimensionality as a parameter of mental functioning.
These concepts refer not so much to a theory of conflict as in
classical metapsychology, but rather to a theory of gradient
which will lead to Meltzer's theory of the aesthetic object.
This book displays brilliantly the creativity of psychoanalytic work applied to a new psychopathological field, both in
helping the patients recover their mental health and also in
understanding new layers of the human mind.

Virginia Ungar (of the Buenos Aires Psychoanalytical Society),
also looking forward to further work on the aesthetic dimension,
writes:

> While we accompany the author on his journey (which he
> says is more like a traveller's tale than a scientific report)
> we can clearly perceive how, alongside the rich and evoca-
> tive clinical descriptions, a complete picture emerges of
> certain modalities of mental functioning. These modalities
> observed in autistic children have a more general scope than
> in psychopathology and even lead us to rethink certain basic
> concepts in psychoanalysis. The research recorded in this
> book allowed Meltzer to come into contact with children
> who were unable to form an object containing a space to be
> used in their mental development. Later, using conclusions
> drawn from this work, Meltzer went on to formulate the
> 'aesthetic conflict' in a book which pairs with this one: *The
> Apprehension of Beauty* (1988).

And Maria Rhode (Tavistock Clinic, London), focussing particularly on language development, says that Meltzer 'was so far
ahead of his time that we are only beginning to realise how he
anticipated recent developmental research ... extending the scope
of psychoanalysis to wide new fields of thought.'

Marisa Pelella Melega (of the Brazilian Psychoanalytical
Society, Sao Paulo) writes of work with a post-autistic patient:

> Donald Meltzer's brilliant 'lessons' supervising my analysis
> of a post-autistic boy have increased my psychoanalytical
> instruments for investigating the transference and coun-
> tertransference: how to observe emotional and behavioural

facts during the session (not only verbalizations), and how to seek out my own dream images in order to carry on with the analysis.

Indeed, Meltzer suggests that it is with the post-autistic child that psychoanalysis comes into its own, with its special capacity to describe hindrances to personality development—which has in a sense not even started with the child locked in autism proper, a mysterious condition for which psychoanalytic terminology offers just one formulation or approach out of many equally valid ones. Hence the book's subtitle: 'A Psychoanalytical Study'.

To conclude, this book documents the basis for a significant expansion of the psychoanalytic model of the mind, going beyond ambivalence to include the mysterious concept of mindlessness (which Meltzer derived from Bion's 'proto-mental', the paradoxical possibility of the mind having a non-mental level of existence): an expansion which is expressed by Meltzer autobiographically as a kind of revelation:

> And so they came together: the key of alpha-function and the lock of two-dimensionality; … The problem area that the key of symbol formation was called into play to open, was the enigma of the inside and the outside of the aesthetic object. Its power to evoke emotionality was only equalled by its ability to generate anxiety, doubt, distrust. While the sensual qualities of the aesthetic object could be apprehended with some degree of confidence, its internal qualities, being infra- or supra-sensual, carried no such comfort. (*Studies in Extended Metapsychology*, 2018 [1976], p. 248)

We need look no further for a plausible explanation of the psychological roots of these highly sensuous children's preference for evasion of the aesthetic conflict entailed in object relations; and what mother could cope with the weight of responsibility devolved in the face of even the slightest mismatch in aesthetic reciprocity?

Meg Harris Williams
(editor)

SECTION A

THEORY

CHAPTER ONE

Aims, scope and methods of the investigation

Donald Meltzer

This small book is not intended as an exhaustive study of a particular pathological syndrome. It is perhaps more like a traveller's tale than a report of scientific inquiry. We can give the compass bearings we followed, the equipment we took and the experience of past travels which served as the basis of our judgments. The rest is all description of the terrain and in habitants, flora and fauna, and the adventures along the way. Furthermore it is all hindsight, for we planned nothing of the sort in advance and only thought to organize ourselves as a group for the purpose of review, and later for the writing up and publication of our experiences.

In fact the children being described in later chapters were among the most interesting of a somewhat larger group of children treated by the psychoanalytical method in private or in clinics over a period from 1960 to 1970. The two items which the various cases had in common were (a) the therapists had all been trained in the psychoanalytical method of child therapy as developed by Melanie Klein; and (b) they all came into supervision from time to time with one of us (D. M.) because he was known to have a special interest in autistic children and to have had some experience of their treatment by the psychoanalytical method. As the clinical work progressed at its own pace and new realizations made their appearance in one child's treatment after another, it began to become apparent that a definitive view of autism was taking shape which differed greatly from anything previously suggested in the literature of psychoanalysis or child psychiatry. The Melanie Klein Trust then gave us a grant to review the experience as a research group in 1967, which injunction we carried out for three years in bi-weekly seminars. The fruits of this work trickled into print in several papers, to a congress of paediatric psychiatry at Rome (D. M.), to the British Psychological Association (D. M.), to the Association of Child Psychotherapists (S. H.), to an international congress of psychoanalysis (D. M.). But the bulk has been fairly laboriously gathered together to form a book which we believe has a very compelling internal logic and sequence.

The scope then of these investigations is narrow indeed. We have carried out some psychoanalytical therapy on various children believed to fall into the general category of Early Infantile Autism, but in very varied stages of evolution. The aim has been a purely descriptive one; to find a language as free from jargon on the one hand and ambiguity on the other to communicate the unusual quality of human relations, view of the world and processes of development presented by these children in the special setting of the psychoanalytical playroom. The method of therapy has been not in any way different from that employed in the treatment of neurotic or psychotic children, as described by Melanie Klein in *The Psychoanalysis of Children* and exemplified in the *Narrative of a Child Analysis*. The core of the method is a systematic and uncompromising investigation of the transference. The material to be described and discussed in later chapters will be seen to owe very little indeed to any other source of information, and certainly the theoretical formulations which we have reached for unifying our descriptions are based entirely upon the observed transactions in the transference between child and analyst.

But it must not be thought that, in speaking of 'description', we claim objectivity; that, in attempting to free our language from jargon, we believe that judgment has been reserved. On the contrary, we would assume that the psychoanalytical method is subjective, introspective, constantly employing differential judgments and based upon a system of preconceptions which embraces the whole life-history of each individual therapist. The position we claim, of having been able to unify, simplify and harmonize these individual experiences, is either quite extraordinary or blatant self-deception. But we do in fact believe that several years of struggle with one another, the material, the inadequacy of language and the near-exotic quality of the children has borne such fruit, enough at least to overcome our trepidation at making the findings public.

Nonetheless it will be a disappointing book to the reader, for it cannot make therapeutic claims or announce a solution to anything. In fact it will soon be clear to a discerning reader that we are in the business of locating problems rather than of solving them. This is probably really the fundamental truth about the human sciences in general and psychoanalysis in particular. Thus we believe we have located some very mysterious phenomena of the mind by recognizing them operative in very condensed form in the children treated. These phenomena, of dismantling, impairment of spatial and temporal concepts, employment of mindlessness as a temporizing move — all these seem to us to throw a very bright beam on modes of thought and relationship discernible elsewhere, in normal or ill people, in the analytic consulting room as in everyday life.

CHAPTER TWO

The psychology of autistic states and of post-autistic mentality

Donald Meltzer

I n this chapter we wish to describe in outline. a formulation of the findings which are subsequently to be described in detail by the individual therapists. We have all been somewhat surprised by the complexity of the ideas which have evolved among us during the years of working together. There can be, of course, no apologizing for such complexity except in so far as we must leave unanswered the question of whether it is a manifestation of our inability to reach simple, more comprehensive, more precise formulations and modes of expression, or whether the complexity does indeed reside in the nature of the material itself.

The main aspect of this complexity is the view which tends to divide the autistic state of mind proper from qualities of mentality in general which appear in these children during the course of development, and are in a sense outside the autism proper - what we see as the residues of the autism. This in itself does not appear to be a very complicated idea, having a rather ordinary medical heritage in the concepts of disease and sequellae; the complexity rather resides in the actual interweaving of the two in any particular child during any particular period of observation. This will be most clearly exemplified in the material of Timmy (J. B.), with whom observations lent themselves to a most convincing mode of study. Over a period of months it became clear that certain forms of behaviour which appeared in great abundance constituted Timmy's autistic phenomena; and by culling out of the record those items which seemed clearly outside this category, and linking them together like pearls on a thread, we were able to construct sequences (sometimes covering several sessions) which could then be interpreted as if they had been indeed quite consecutive. The result was something akin to the cinematic photography of the blossoming of flowers, taken at one frame every few minutes, in which the balletic unfolding and growth describes a pattern unseen by the waking eye.

But perhaps even more important than the individual revelation about Timmy was the assurance we gained from this observation regarding the degree of isolation in which the two categories of phenomena were held in the child's mind. It is of course no great novelty that different parts of the mind should be held at a distance, implying non-recognition of one another; this is a commonplace aspect of repression, splitting processes, delusional systems. But what appeared as a great novelty and as a dazzling display of the speed and complexity of the mental apparatus, was the way in which the two categories of phenomena were interwoven and interdigitated. In this   juxtaposition of mental states the autistic phenomena could be seen to stand in the same relation to the transference material as do ordinary play disruptions in child analysis. But while a play disruption involves a switch to a different level or aspect of the transference situation, the autistic disruption gave quite a different impression; it seemed more like the intrusion of a petit mal attack into the conversation: as if, had these been talking processes, the sentence interrupted would have been subsequently completed, once the autistic 'noise' ceased. A much older child, Barry (D. W.), developed a pattern of sleeping in the session which gave much the same impression of suspended mental functioning.

The point about this suspension of the transactions in the transference is that it gradually appeared to us to be the key to the comprehension of the central problem in autism: namely the quality of the autistic state, and its special impingement on personality development. The problem of finding language with which to describe our realization of this state is quite insurmountable if we are to avoid a tautological coil of words that would gradually tighten into a strangling knot of jargon.

The autistic state of mind

Let us, as Whitehead (*Adventures of Ideas,* 1933) suggests, think of past, present and future in its most immediate form stretching over the miniscule gulf of (say) two-tenths of a second: now, one-tenth of a second ago, one-tenth of a second to come. Consider life to be posting ahead on this wave-like motion, the present being forwarded like the surf-rider on the crest of revolving events as the present moment passes into recollection and the anticipated moment arrives to sustain the present experience. This present moment would be non-existent, crushed between past and future, achieving merely a precarious psychic reality in the organization of recollection. It would be truly retrospective, even if only by one-tenth of a second.

If we then conceive this thread of time to have strung upon it those pearls of recollection of which we have already spoken, we may tentatively take mental life to be so defined as to differentiate it from the linear sequence of neuro-physiological events in the brain, concrete, disparate, joined end-to-end. Mental events would thus stand in relation to neurophysiological ones in a logical way akin to that of a frequency modulation to its carrier band, as a model. Such a model is fairly central to any conception of the autistic process proper which will view it as essentially a suspension of mental life. By delineating it in this manner, we place its events outside the stream of aggregated and, eventually, organized recollection. Comparing it with the event of a petit mal attack suggests the possibility of neurophysiological factors, which we would wish to leave open for investigation by other methods; our psychoanalytical method, which depends so heavily upon the observation and interpretation of the transference, can make nothing of the longitudinal content of the autistic state proper. But of course, like any other observer of behaviour, we are in a position to formulate some cross-sectional concept of its structure and dynamics. This formulation, which we now wish to present in outline, will be exemplified particularly in the clinical material of Timmy (J.B.), but its details have been drawn from two sources: the first is that already mentioned, namely direct observation of the autistic phenomena; the second, to which we owe much of the conviction we feel about the first type of data, is a reconstructive matter: *by recognising the qualities of mind which are peculiar to the states and functioning of such children outside the realm of the autism proper, we are able to see, separately deployed, several tendencies which, when exercised in a consortium, produce the autistic state.*

What then are the mental tendencies that we would list as characteristic and, in that sense, prerequisite to the appearance of autism as a pathological condition? It will become apparent that such a descriptive undertaking, however determined to stay within the confines of metapsychology, soon finds itself in such a misty and boggy landscape that it runs out of well established technical terms, and is forced back upon a mixture of poetic description and philosophic abstraction. What we will try to do above all, is to avoid neologism and pseudo-precision. For the sake of psychoanalytic tidiness, we will discuss the factors under the headings of economics, structure, dynamics and genetics.

Economic factors

The children studied appear to us to be highly intelligent. What do we mean by this, and how have we reached such an assessment? Their mental processes operate at great speed. Even when dominated by repetitiveness, the rapidity with which new combinations and permutations of the same basic configuration of phantasy are evolved, is quite dazzling. Their accessibility to sensory data both from the body and from the outside world gives the impression of an apparatus naked to the wind. Consequently their discrimination of the details of the environment and of alterations in these details is quite intimidating. The complexity of their mental functioning taxes the therapist at every point. Added to this there is a subtlety of emotive response and sensitivity to the mental and physical state of the therapist which far exceeds that encountered in child analysis generally, and certainly is in quite a different category from the atmosphere of the adult consulting-room.

Added to this intelligence and the factors of perceptual sensitivity connected with it, the children present an emotional sensibility which we would wish to describe as a kind of gentleness of disposition. Their awareness of the mental states of the person to whom they feel intimately related does seem to contain a predilection for depressive concern that is not the same as identification; it is in the nature of a primitive permeability to the emotions of others – another aspect of the 'nakedness' mentioned above. But it is clear that they also tend to experience their objects as similarly permeable and likely to be bombarded with awareness of the pain of others; and evidence to the contrary would seem to be interpreted by them as tokens of rejection rather than as signs of incapacity in the object.

This tendency to be bombarded by awareness of the pain in others, coupled with the inclination to interpret emotional obtuseness in others as rejection, makes for a very special vulnerability to catastrophic modes of depressive experience; this will be most clearly seen in the material of John (I. W.).

The likelihood that this liability to depressive pain is related to the special nakedness to the emotional winds emanating from others seems further suggested by the very minimal intensity of persecutory anxiety to be observed. This would also link with the impression of gentleness of disposition, given in terms of minimal sadism: for what often appears as a ruthless cruelty to 'the mother's other babies' is not dictated by sadism seizing upon rivalry as the justification for its expression, but does rather emerge in the service of an uncompromising possessiveness of the maternal object. The autistic children wish unequivocally to be rid of all rivals, for every deprivation or disappointment seems to be directly experienced in this framework. They are not particularly intent upon inflicting pain, nor is sadistic glee a prominent feature of their emotionality. While triumph is a regular ingredient of their pleasures, its quality is predominantly joyous rather than sadistic, until splitting-and-idealization becomes established in the post-autistic development.

This joyous possession of the maternal object constitutes a primitive form of love which is both tender and highly sensual. The surface, skin-to-skin intimacy they seek, tends to be in satiable and to resent, and resist, the impact of time. It is from this factor, rather than from either the inroads of persecutory anxiety or the importunate thrust of raw instinct, that the children's strong compulsion to repetition appears to arise.

This rather impressive list of dispositional items, all contributing to the economic tendencies of the personality, appears to us to be ubiquitous within the group, and may even be taken as prerequisite. To recapitulate, the factors are: high intelligence, sensitivity to the emotional state of others, liability to depressive pain of a massive sort, minimal sadism and consequently minimal persecution; possessive jealousy; the children are highly sensual in their love, and prone to endless time-arresting repetition of the joy and triumph of possession.

Structural characteristics

As we have indicated, we are taking the view that the autistic state proper can be separated from the states of mind in the same child which reside outside the autism. The ways in which the one influences the other will be described later. At this point we must face the difficult task of trying to define a structure of the autism proper, which is both a mental one, and yet at the same time is essentially mindless. And as we have said, the key to the situation is seen to lie in the temporary suspension of the recognition of time passing; but it is something quite different from the various types of denial of time, the circular concept, the oscillating concept, or fragmented time of other sorts. We wish to envisage a structure, the ego–id–superego-ideal, being dismantled in a manner that has the following qualities: it must be accomplished in a moment; it must be reversible almost effortlessly, as if drawn once more together by the inertia of mental springs; its transactions must be of a quality which disqualifies them from linkage with other mental events. To express this latter quality, we would like to make a distinction between 'event' and 'experience', assuming that 'events' are discrete, unavailable for linkage and thus fundamentally unavailable for recollection.

The events, then, which represent themselves in the forms of behaviour described by us as the phenomenology of the autistic state proper, do not lend themselves to apprehension by the child as experiences, with their characteristic structure of the infinitesimal point of the present compressed between recollection and anticipation. How does this take place? We have employed above the term 'dismantling', to which we must now give precise significance in order to differentiate it from splitting processes.

These latter processes are understood to employ destructive impulses in order to make attacks on linking. These attacks are, in the main, directed primarily against objects, and have only a secondary consequence of splitting the ego, or, more correctly, the self. This secondary splitting seems to be a consequence of the division in the object, much in the way that a split in the territory of a disputed region between two contending nations would galvanize a polarization of the population involved: being confronted by a split in the object, incompatible loyalties within the self causes it to fall into similar (in the geometric sense) bits. It is for this reason that the primal splitting-and idealization of the object is prerequisite to the division between good and bad in the self and its impulses.

We envisage 'dismantling' as a very different sort of process with very different implications. In the first place it seems to us to occur in a passive rather than an active way, somewhat akin to allowing a brick wall to fall to pieces by the action of weather, moss, fungi and insects, through failing to point it with mortar. Dismantling occurs by a passive device of allowing the various senses, both special and general, internal and external, to attach themselves to the most stimulating object of the moment. It would be a mere coincidence if the most highly coloured, arrestingly shaped, most odoriferous, noisiest, tastiest, softest, warmest sensations of the moment, were all emanating from the same real external object. Except for the baby at the breast, such sensa are highly likely to be emanated by a variety of objects at any one moment; and with the exception of the most charismatic objects of art or qualities of personality, most objects have attention 'paid' to them. We are inclined to experience this deployment within ourselves as an active process. It is uncertain whether Western man has, in general, retained the capacity to suspend attention, as the yogi guru claims to do through extreme concentration on nothingness. What we usually call 'inattention' is really wandering of attention, either in the sense of diminished focus, or turning inward in rumination or daydream.

We are suggesting, then, the existence of some capacity (whose mechanism we will attempt to investigate later) for suspending attention, which allows the senses to wander, each to its most attractive object of the moment. This scattering seems to bring about the dismantling of the self as a mental apparatus, but in a very passive, falling-to-bits way. There are toys which represent a dog (say), made of wooden beads and held together by strings which pass through holes in a board and are fastened to a ring. A child holding the little board with his finger in the ring can make the dog stand up by exerting a tension on the ring, or allow him to collapse into a reclining posture by relaxing the tension; and we are envisaging attention as the strings which hold the senses together in consensuality. This 'common sense' as Bion wryly calls it, apprehends objects in the multifaceted way which is essential to mental acts, as opposed to neurophysiological events. We are employing a structural concept of attention which is similar to Freud's delineation of consciousness as a mental 'organ'.

If this is a reasonable approximation of the process that induces the autistic state, namely that by suspending attention the child is able to let his mental organization fall passively to pieces, it would seem quite certain that neither persecutory anxiety nor despair would result from this mode of withdrawal from the world, since violence to neither self nor object is in involved. This implies that the reinstatement of the pre-existing organization would have no gradient of mental pain (Bion's Ps↔D) to overcome. A social equivalent to it would be, for instance, the famous story about 'Captain' Abraham Lincoln as a young man during the Black Hawk War of 1832, as told by Carl Sandburg: 'As their captain was drilling them one day with two platoons advancing toward a gate, he couldn't think of the order that would get them endwise, two by two, for passing through the gate. So he commanded, "This company is dismissed for two minutes, when it will fall in again on the other side of the gate".'

Dynamic aspects

Our idea then is that the sensory components of the self, which have been dismantled in order to pass through the autistic 'gate', can also effortlessly 'fall in' on the other side. By now we have probably multiplied our models beyond any gain in clarity, and will profit more by turning to the dynamics of the process. Here we are confronted with the compulsive tendency which is so marked in these children, and find ourselves surprised to discover certain primitive aspects of compulsivity which are not easily discernible in more sophisticated forms of employment. The most arresting feature of compulsivity generally is the repetitiveness of the act, or thought underlying it, in a potentially endless series, which then, as mysteriously as it commenced, comes to rest. Investigation of the neuroses has shown us clearly the factors operative within it; how omnipotent separation and control of objects induces either. persecutory or depressive anxiety, depending on the degree of cruelty in the motivation. The compulsive repetition can be seen to express the need for repeated monitoring of the objects because of their tendency to reunite; and on the other hand it expresses the necessity of serving and nurturing them, since the separating (by interfering with processes of reparation) tends to result in dilapidation.

Thus an interplay of primary and secondary motives of defence against anxiety is evident in obsessional states. This emphasis on the role of defence against anxiety, oedipal in the first place and then persecutory or depressive, results in a picture of compulsivity as a mechanism of defence but obscures its more primitive roots in the repetition compulsion. What Freud could refer to as the timelessness of the system-unconscious (uncs.) in his earlier period of formulation, the 'topographic', would need to be referred to the id in 'structural' theory. Apprehension of time is certainly an ego-function, as we have already described at some length. The compulsion to repeat is the overriding economic principle of the id, as the pleasure-pain-reality principle is of the ego in its relation to id and external world, and as the paranoid-schizoid-depressive positions are in the ego's relation to superego-ideal.

Freud's investigation of the compulsion to repeat, as undertaken in 'Beyond the pleasure principle', is perhaps too speculative and cosmological to be of immediate use in clinical investigation. A more neurophysiological grounding of our conception is required. It is when we attempt to comprehend the nature of the id that psychoanalysis makes its rapprochement with work in other fields of psychology such as conditioning of reflexes, the perceptual processes studied by the Gestalt school, ethological studies and neuropathology. When the self is dismantled into its sensual components by the suspension of the ego-function of attention, a coherent ego ceases temporarily to exist; each fragment, or rather component, is reduced to a primitive state dominated by the id and its economics and dynamics. This primitiveness is, we suggest, essentially mindless. Its events cannot be considered as mental acts, and they cannot be experienced in any way which allows for integration in the continuum of recollection, nor as a basis for anticipation.

But the mystery that appears in the study of compulsivity in the neurotic, namely what circumstances can terminate the potentially endless repetition, does find some tentative answer in the observation of autistic states proper. Both John (I. W.) and Timmy (J. B.) illustrate very clearly the high degree of sensual apprehension of the therapist which characterized the transference relationship. It became apparent fairly early on in our work that it was necessary for the therapist to be able to *mobilize the suspended attention of the child in its autistic state, in order to bring it back into transference contact.* To this end, continual interpretation was required, of the transference-state before the lapse into autism, along with more intuitively learned techniques of voice employment, attentiveness, and posture. The latter included a degree of permissiveness with regard to physical contact, in touching, looking, smelling and tasting, that one would not easily allow in the course of child analysis ordinarily.

This direct bodily availability of the therapist seemed to have its charismatic effect because of the overwhelming oral sensuality of the children. Timmy (J. B.) would put his mouth near the talking mouth of the therapist and concretely eat the emerging language. John (I. W.) would look into his therapist's eyes or down her jumper exactly as he peered through the glass rose of the window on the stairway. The breast significance of the therapist as a part-object in the transference became established early in the treatment and in a primitive sensual way, long before it could be seen to take on a more abstract significance; and of course surprisingly early compared with the long and difficult struggle toward it in the course of analysis of the neurotic patient, adult or child.

Genetic considerations

In short, it could be said that the maternal breast, as an object of high consensual attractiveness, seemed to function as the magnet or spring to draw together the dismantled self by commanding, one might even say commandeering, the attention. The autistic 'attack' could be seen to terminate by this sort of springing together of the self, which allowed the child then to continue the transference activity that had been temporarily suspended. It can well be imagined that the drift into autism as a developmental disturbance has a fine economic relation to the intensity of the breast relationship to the mothering person. When this withers, as it probably does when depression or other disturbance in the mother dries up her attentiveness, warmth, chatter and sensuality toward the baby, the dismantled self will tend to float away for longer and longer periods of mindless activity. It is conceivable that the degree of arrest in the development might well have a near arithmetic relation to the waking, and perhaps the sleeping, life-time spent in the state of autism proper. The therapeutic and prophyllactic implications of this are obvious. To this quantitative factor, must be added the effects upon development when those same tendencies which make the autistic state possible are not employed in consortium but more singly in the course of life experience and object relations. In this area we have learned most from the treatment of Piffie (S. H.) and Barry (D. W.).

Personality development in the autistic child

Formulations of the autistic state proper, such as the one above, cannot claim (as we have said) any methodological priority over other methods of observation or other systems of formulation. While the observations have been carried out in the analytical setting by analytically trained workers, they suffer as much from the limitations of that setting and training as they can be said to profit from it. But when we enter upon a description and formulation of the personality development of these children outside the autism proper, and in a sense post-autistic with Barry (D. W.) and Piffie (S. H.), we can claim to speak with the special insight that the analytic method alone, we believe, can afford in these matters. This special authority pertains, of course, only to the unconscious structure, dynamics and economics of the mind, and the special (and one-sided) view of personality genesis they make available.

We have already spoken of the general quantitative consideration, namely the loss of maturational mental lifetime which is replaced by autistic states proper. We must now turn to the specific interferences with development and the consequences that can be traced with the psychoanalytical method. These fall into two large categories: interferences with the achievement of personality structure, and the obsessional eccentricity of object relations. These two will later be exemplified in the clinical descriptions of Barry (D. W.) and Piffie (S. H.) respectively. In the theoretical formulation here we will stress the operation of unconscious phantasy in the children, since it is to this that our method of investigation gives us insights of a first order of validity. Just how these operations in the child dovetail with personality tendencies in the mothering person or in the organization of the nurturing milieu, we will leave for discussion in the final summing-up of the investigations, since it is reconstructive and therefore of a secondary order of validity.

Personality structure has two dimensions that go beyond the delineation of id, ego and superego as described by Freud. Indeed, this categorization has a certain biological validity which is somewhat different from the one which appears as the functional organization: namely the division into self and objects. In addition to this functional division, we can discern a second order of structuring relating to the organization of the life space: namely the geography of personality in its four characteristic regions – internal and external to the self, inside and outside of objects. The fifth area, the 'nowhere' of the delusional system, does not concern us here. Of these two general dimensions of personality structure, organization of the geography of the life-space and organization of the self and objects, the former appears to be of primary significance in the psycho pathology of the post-autistic personality (as we will henceforth call it, meaning both outside the autistic states proper and the sequellae of Early Infantile Autism).

(a) Organization of the life-space

We are inclined to think that the yield in understanding of the beginnings of the life of the mind is particularly rich in this realm of study with autistic children, revealing processes which are indeed so primitive as to be quite inaccessible to other methods or with other types of patient. These children seem to suffer from an absolute hindrance to progress in development because of difficulty in differentiating these four areas in the geography of phantasy. They experience a geographic type of confusion which far outstrips in complexity that induced by massive projective identification. How does it come about? Or perhaps the more correct question is the converse one: Why does the ordinary differentiation not come about? The answer we can offer is fairly complicated.

In order to explain this failure we must return to the disposition of the children, in particular to their high degree of orality, their intense possessive jealousy of the maternal object, their primitive sensuality and their tender, non-sadistic makeup, all of which disposes them to early and intense depressive experiences. The sensuality and possessiveness induce a strong trend towards fusion with their object, which is easily recognized in the playroom by such acts as burrowing into the therapist, appropriating the therapist's hands to accomplish manipulations, demanding to use the therapist's body as if it were furniture. But the very insistence upon control over the therapist's body reveals the failure to achieve any degree of projective identification. This surprising fact, and the extraordinary behaviour which makes it manifest, pertains just as well to the room, the house, underneath the table or inside the cupboard. The child cannot for any length of time experience the distinction between being inside and being outside the object. Looking into the therapist's eyes can be immediately transformed into looking out of the window. But the moment of triumph over (say) the birds in the garden as the excluded outside-babies, immediately turns into enraged fist-shaking and banging the head on the window, and then to burrowing and banging the head on the therapist's chest. The outside-babies have suddenly turned into the triumphant inside-babies, and the triumph of the child turns to puzzled rage.

One child showed us the answer in a single stroke of creative intensity. For months he had drawn doors and gates, usually with complex wrought-iron grills. Then gradually rather Victorian gothic houses took shape. One day he painstakingly drew an ornate house seen from the front on one side of the page, a house in Northwood, while on the other side he drew a back view of a pub in Southend. Thus the child demonstrated his experience of a two-dimensional object; when you enter by the front door you simultaneously exit by the rear door of a different object. It is in effect an object without an inside.

But how does such an object come into existence? To answer this one has to reconsider the extremely insistent intrusiveness of these children in respect of the maternal object, and the way in which the primitive sensuality permits an easy shifting between animate and inanimate objects, much in the way that Winnicott's transitional objects arise – a subject which we will return to in the final summing-up. This easy substitution, even outside the autism proper, even when objects are being consensually apprehended, does support the omnipotence of the intrusive phantasies. In effect, as we shall see in Barry's material, the maternal object is experienced as patent, its orifices unprotected, devoid of sphincters, open to the weather and the marauder alike. Like 'Tintern Abbey', the distinction between inside and outside is not a fact, only an idea constructed by the imagination. It is of course tempting to think that these children have been exposed to some extraordinary degree of maternal preoccupation in their early months, the in-one-ear-and-out-the-other type of 'yes, dear' attention. Occasionally the history of severe depression in the mother post-partum seems to bear this out. But we are more inclined to seek the solution of the puzzle in the child himself, for surely every baby and child gets quite a lot of 'yes, dear'-ing from busy mothers.

No, the transactions of the playroom strongly suggest that the insistent intrusiveness, the promiscuous sensuality and the intense possessiveness incline these children to experience an absolute possession of an unpossessable object, rich in surface qualities but devoid of substance, a paper-thin object without a delineated inside. This produces a primal failure of the containing function of the external object, and thus of the formation of the concept of self as a container. This serious defect does not seem to be precisely the same as that described by Bick as an inadequate skin for the self, since that does not appear to involve any deficiency of concept formation, but rather an inadequate function of containing under stress of anxiety. We do not see the characteristic spilling-out of parts of the self nor the secondary skin function that she has so clearly described.

On the contrary our impression is that the internal spacelessness of self and object in the post-autistic personality is a continuous defect unrelated to stress of anxiety. It also appears to have a differential relation to the various sensory modalities in keeping with the general tendency to looseness of consensual function. The weakest of these modalities, as regards containment, would appear to be the auditory one, with special regard to the language function. 'In-one-ear-and-out-the-other' seems, very concretely, to be the case. It is in this area of defect that we are inclined to look for an explanation of the apparent deafness which so often first attracts attention and arouses alarm in the parents. The relation of this to the mutism is, however, a more complex problem whose detailed consideration must wait.

This deficiency of containment related to internal spacelessness of the self produces a type of manic quality in the personality, which will be seen very clearly in John and Timmy. The inability to retain objects has an effect equivalent to the sadistic expulsion of them as faeces as seen in the manic disorders, but with a somewhat helpless, automatic quality that is quite distinctive and can suddenly result in the catastrophic depressive collapse into desperate sobbing. The material concerning Timmy's 'squeezing' will illustrate the struggle of the child to close his own orifices. But the child's openness is not only confined to the difficulty in retaining mental and therefore also physical contents. We are inclined to see these children as suffering also from a sensory openness which is experienced as a bombardment of sensa. This bombardment appears to com pound the difficulty in retaining, and renders the ordinary process of working over in phantasy (and therefore probably in dreaming) relatively inefficient for play, and thus for learning. The consequence of this is a*n unusual degree of dependence upon the mental functions, and not merely upon the services, of an external object.*

This consideration, we think, accounts for much of the mental-defective-like quality in these highly intelligent children. Perhaps it would be worthwhile to elaborate a bit on this point, as it has important implications both for understanding the nature of the post-autistic personality and for guiding any therapeutic approach. Freud considered thought to be an economic form of trial action. When our internal equipment fails to cope with the complexity of representations involved in a problem, we have recourse to counters – an abacus, a chess board and pieces, paper and pencil and geometer's instruments, for example. In the same way a child uses toys, as counters for the objects of phantasy and thought. When the counters take on a life of their own and a value apart from that assigned in the representation, we say that the play or game has become concrete and that a failure of symbol formation is manifest.

The post-autistic personality does of course, along with all primitive states, present a degree of concreteness in thought and phantasy. But in fact this is not seen to nearly the high degree that the gross immaturity would lead one to expect. Instead one sees a somewhat more complicated process which involves *the employment of the maternal object (or object of maternal transference) as an extension of the self for the performance of ego-functions.* Where another child would climb onto the windowsill, John would simply make anticipatory movements to be lifted; when Piffie could not hold all the pieces and figures in his hand he naturally deposited them in the therapist's lap. In order to make toys disappear when they had become tainted by suspicion of having been handled by other children, Timmy would deposit them under the therapist's chair, as if leaving rubbish for the dustmen. Other children would have arranged a place of safekeeping or thrown the toys in the dustbin.

The point is that it was natural for these children to experience the situation as calling for the therapist to perform an ego-function. He had to function not merely as a servant or surrogate, but as a prime mover in the situation; he was not only to carry out the action, but also to decide what action was to be taken, and therefore to carry the responsibility. In this sense the child could be said to act with a politic type of incapacity, like an oriental potentate who knows nothing of the methods of tax collection, but is ready to behead his vizeer if injustice is revealed. The question arises regarding the relation of this type of dependence to omnipotence and omnipotent control over objects. We would suggest that the two processes are very different and can be seen to be active in very different ways in these children, the latter as an aspect of the obsessionality and the former as a special type of dependence.

Where the therapist's disobedience in respect of tyrannical control brings a fairly ordinary reaction of rage, failure to perform the required ego function for the child produces bewilderment and a tendency to withdraw into the Autistic State Proper. It is a clear indication also that the autistic states proper are not to be understood as derived by mechanisms of defence against anxiety, but tend to be brought about by bombardment of sensa in the face of both inadequate equipment and failure of dependence.

This naturally gives rise to the question of the relation between the post-autistic personality and the personality of the first month of life. In this area we are, of course, only conjecturing, but it would appear a cogent guess that the quality of the dependence seen in the post-autistic state is very akin indeed to that of the newborn, in that it is dependent upon the object for both services and ego-functions. This implies a narcissistic bond which not only extends the body of the child into the more capable one of the object, but also extends the mind itself. This would therefore suggest a process far more related to the identification Freud described as characteristic of primary narcissism, and so have a very different quality from, say, the confusion of self and object due to projective identification. In the latter type of operation, the child's mind and body take over, in all the limitations of ego-functioning characteristic of the infantile ego. It is for this reason that the pseudo-mature behaviour pursuant to projective identification is merely a childish caricature of adult conduct.

If we conceive of this type of dependence in the sense of primary narcissism and recollect Freud's statement that in the earliest times relationship and identification are quite indistinguishable, we are led back to the problem of the two dimensional quality of object and of self in the autistic child's personality structure. Bion's conception of maternal reverie as a process in which the mother takes in the disturbed part of the infant's personality, divests it of distress and then returns it to the child, would seem a very unifying and clarifying idea here; but we would need to see it functioning in a somewhat different way from ordinary maternal care. In the first place these children would appear to require the mother to take in, contain and divest of pain the child entire, not merely a part; and because of this, and perhaps because of other limiting aspects of the mother's state of mind, a primal failure of dependence occurs. This, we feel, is experienced by the child as the paper-thin mother or breast.

As we probably cannot usefully elaborate further on these points until the clinical material is before us, we will turn our attention now to the second dimension of personality structuring and its disturbance in the post-autistic organization.

(b) Organization of the self and objects

It has been suggested that the study of the organization of the life space in these children gives a high yield of scientific information about the very earliest process in this area; and a similar reward may be gained from the study of the organization of self and objects. But it is of a more restricted sort: namely that we discover phenomena related to the primitive aspects of obsessional mechanisms which are both of general interest with regard to obsessionality, and of very specific interest concerning the obsessional element in the perversions and especially the position of the fetishistic plaything, as the editor (D. M.) has described elsewhere (*Sexual States of Mind*, 1973).

We take the point of view that obsessionality may be described in general as arising from two factors in the relation of self to objects: first of all, it depends on omnipotent control over the objects; and secondly, it relies on attacks on linking to separate the objects in order that they may be better controlled. Although it seems that the logical order of the operations is as stated

– control first followed by separation to bulwark control – we wish to discuss the two in the converse order.

As stated earlier, we find that these children have to a high degree the capacity to dissociate their sensory modalities from their ordinary consensual linkage to one another. We are inclined to view this ordinary function in the light of Bion's formulation of alpha-function, as a way of describing the mental function which makes sensa available as thoughts for manipulation in thinking. We wish to describe another kind of failure which produces sensual events which are only suitable for enjoyment, and cannot be apprehended as experiences either for manipulation in thinking or, therefore, for communication. We think these events differ from Bion's 'beta elements' which are suitable only for evacuation.

While in its extreme form this dissociation of consensuality is found to be the essential operation for the formation of the autistic state proper, its partial usage is characteristic of the post-autistic personality and is the basis of the extreme obsessionality, as will be exemplified in the material of Piffie. Again we must stress that the attack on linking is directed against the ego and is very passive and non-sadistic in its mode. The ego function of attention is manipulated in a way that simply allows the experience of objects to fall to bits, and to spring back together.

This differentiation, between direct destructive attacks upon the links between objects or part-objects, and indirect attacks upon such links through dismantling the self's capacity for consensual experience, does seem to us to be an important general distinction with regard to obsessional disorders. The great mystery about these disorders has always been the wide degree of variation in the degree of persecutory anxiety consequent to the establishment of omnipotent control and separation of objects. In general, of course, one has realized that the degree of persecution consequent to the operation of a defence was proportional to the degree of sadism with which it was mounted. Freud, in his papers 'On fetishism' (1927) and 'Splitting of the ego in the process of defence' (1938) showed the way towards the solving of this mystery, which he correctly linked with the general problem of the maintenance of mental health in the face of unresolved infantile conflicts. Melanie Klein's further investigation of splitting processes in her 1946 paper 'A note on some schizoid mechanisms' and in later contributions, pursued the problem of psychopathology primarily. We can now add substance of a certain precision to Freud's formulation of the operation of splitting processes in the service of preserving the healthy part of the personality from encroachment and from subservience (as it were) to the ill parts.

The process of dismantling the self, especially in its capacity for consensual perceptual experience and therefore its capacity for the introjection of integrated objects, provides a very satisfactory answer to the problem. It was not, after all, merely a question of how health and illness can exist side by side in the same personality without destroying the sanity. The problem was of a more delicate and economic nature: how could good objects be held under control and in a state of separation without so weakening them and thus rendering them vulnerable to sadistic attack from the destructive parts of the personality, as in catatonia? The same principle is used, for instance, in the distinction between binding together a group through concrete links (as in a chain-gang) or abstract ones (as in a secret society), and simply associating the members for the purpose of recognition by themselves and others (as in the case of uniforms of all sorts). The latter method defines the group in terms of recognition – that is, perceptually – rather than in terms of action either imposed or curtailed. Actually in the formation of groups in the outside world both methods are used together – as, for example, with clerical dress and holy vows. It is a continuation or extrapolation of the process in nature whereby species identify themselves to one another and mark off their predators. The mice in the fable wished to put a bell on the cat in order to be able to track its whereabouts; that is, they wished to use their distant perception to identify a predator. Conversely, they would choose a contact percipient to identify the most intimate relationship. This is the general method in nature, to establish distant criteria for the recognition of enemies and proximal ones for the indications of friendship and love. It is just this system that is taken to bits in the dismantling, and by so doing much adaptive capacity is sacrificed.

Just how, then, does the dismantling of the perceptual self affect omnipotent control over objects without weakening them *vis à vis* the destructive parts? Let us suppose, for instance, that the mummy wears a uniform and the daddy wears a bell, so that they are identified by sight and sound respectively. The allocation of the perceptual capacity when dismantled affects the experience as if the child were dealing not with mummy-in-uniform and daddy-with-a-bell, but with deaf-mummy and blind-daddy. Mummy cannot hear daddy's bell and daddy cannot see mummy's uniform. They will pass like the proverbial ships in the night. That is, they will pass the night of the child's discontent well separated in the child's mind.

The important point about such operations is that they result in introjection of defective objects from the point of view of intimate relations. The sexuality built upon such a foundation bends heavily towards the fetishistic, or, to keep to our analogy, in search of a woman with a bell or a man with a uniform. This in fact is precisely what happens in fetishism proper, and contributes the fetishistic element to the object choice throughout the whole range of the perversions.

In the post-autistic personality it manifests itself in the special degree and type of obsessionality which will be described particularly in the material about Piffie. There it will be seen how the preoccupation with keeping the objects incommunicado (as in the episode of the man-on-the-ladder), promotes also a ruminative quasi-scientific curiosity about how things are pieced together and kept from falling apart. One of the most impressive examples of this was in Piffie's period of experimentation with permutations of colour and form in a rather stylized picture of house and tree. Blue sky, green grass, yellow house, red roof, brown tree, etc. Similarly the colour permutations were alternated with the inside and outside of the house. The final impression was that Piffie had no conviction that the blueness of the sky or greenness of the grass was any more essential than the redness of the roof or yellowness of the house, or that if one were inside the house it might not all be reversed. We could see that a certain tyrannical attitude would not brook the blueness of the sky being forever mated to the greenness of the grass, but asserted that this arrangement was under the child's control, that it existed as such only insofar as he saw it so. In the same way in which he could deal with the surprise of the man-on-the-ladder by a series of drawings in which the man gradually ceased to exist as a recollected experience, so he could deal with the everyday facts of nature by selectively employing his sensorium to suit himself. This is an indication of the high intelligence that can employ attention to make such abstractions in the post-autistic state and yet that, when taken to its extreme of non-attention in the autistic state, may appear to be defective.

The obsessionality of character in the post-autistic personality is therefore compounded, one might say, of the tendency to employ dismantling of the self in a particular way for the sake of experiencing omnipotent control and separation of objects, and consequently, of a ruminative preoccupation with the way in which the elements of the world are linked together. To call it quasi-scientific in essence does not belittle the possibility of scientific activity resulting from it in later life. In all likelihood many scientists have had an autistic beginning and a post-autistic character. The natural extrapolation of the post-autistic character would build an idiot-savant way of life; and this tendency can certainly be seen in Piffie and Barry. Another child, whose material could not be included here, had already gone very far along this road, being almost exclusively preoccupied with painting flowers at the age of eight. Robert was fairly ineducable in other areas but in his narcissistic identification with his mother, who was a portrait painter, he did in fact in the most skilled, rapid, organized way, produce quite breathtakingly beautiful water-colours of flowers, precisely coloured and fairly bursting with life.

Our general conclusion, regarding the implications of these findings in autistic children for our understanding of the wider field of obsessionality – in character and neurosis as well as in the compulsive aspect of perversion – is that a spectrum of sadism can be constructed. At one end of this spectrum we would place the extreme of cruel pleasure with which objects are held in a state of suspended animation in catatonia. At the other end would be the non-sadistic dismantling of the self in the post-autistic personality. The one places the objects in a state of torturous enslavement, while the other merely unhinges the capacity of the objects to find one another for intimate contact, inflicting neither pain nor debility. Between these two poles one could arrange the spectrum of obsessional disorders in terms of the relative admixture of these two operations, so as to construct a sort of periodic table referrable to the severity of the mental disorder. It must be remembered that the severity of illness in the post-autistic state is not specially related to the degree of obsessionality, but rather to the other area of the psycho-pathology, namely the disorder in the organization of the life-space and the consequent severe impediment to maturation. The obsessionality is not so much psychopathological as non-adaptive, in the sense that many philosophical or theological systems are non-adaptive if taken as a guide to action in the world. The trouble lies in the interference with emotional responsiveness to the complexity of the world when the 'cerebral' oversimplification of obsessional thought obtrudes upon experience. In a philosophic sense, the aesthetic of the turbulent harmony of growth is sacrificed for the peaceful harmony of order. It is conducive of a state of mind suitable for old age, for recollection of experience, employed at a time of life when there are as yet too few experiences to recall. It produces a Wordsworthian tranquillity at a time of life when turbulent pugnacity is required. Thus Barry, seeking employment and lodgings at the age of 21, could find nothing to meet his requirements, and tended to remain at home as his mother's housekeeper. The possibility that the world might have requirements of him which he should struggle to meet, was simply alien to his mind, much like Melville's Bartleby.

Before closing this introductory survey of the findings which are to be exemplified in the following chapters about the individual children, we might say a few words about the relation of the special type of obsessionality to the problem of so-called transitional objects. In later writings Winnicott recognized the very equivocal value of these constructions: that, while they might indeed serve economically to tide over a child's transition in its object relations, there was great danger of the transitional object taking on a fetishistic significance and being used as a focus for the isolation of a perverse tendency. We feel that the mechanism of dismantling is in fact the basis for the formation of a transitional object. It can be seen to arise in the case of John and his Teddy. But it is also clear that Teddy came gradually to be the focus of organization of the narcissism in which John took refuge from depressive feelings as his autistic tendency lessened. The same happened with Timmy. It was present to a marked degree in Barry's relation to the television machine. Our conclusion is that the formation of a transitional object is in fact an operation most hazardous for personality development, and that its outcome rests very delicately in the balance, depending mainly on the way in which it is greeted by external objects. If the relief of dependence upon the mother, for instance, is too readily accepted by her, the stage is likely to be set for the formation of a strong narcissistic organization involving an essentially perverse use of the transitional object as a fetishistic plaything.

Summary

In this theoretical introduction to the main body of the book, the clinical description of the work with the children, we have tried to present an organized framework of thought within which to catch and order the dazzling display of apparently disparate clinical phenomena. It is meant to save the reader from having to experience quite the degree of confusion and helplessness that we ourselves went through, while hoping not to impose upon him a rigid code of interpretation that might stifle his own freedom of thought.

In essence we have drawn a distinction between the Autistic State Proper (let us now capitalize it as a distinct entity) and the post-autistic development with its special impediments and equally special potentialities. We suggested that the impairment in development due to the operation of Autistic States Proper had a nearly arithmetic relation to the amount of life-time actually involved and distinguished this from the degree of immaturity and character pathology in the post-autistic development. The latter was seen to be dependent upon the interaction of the child's particular tendencies, especially its obsessionality and impairment of dimensionality in object relations, and those of the most important figures of the nurturing environment. On the contrary we are inclined to think that the operation of the consortium of factors which make for the Autistic State Proper is far more intrinsic to the child and only modified by environmental 'failure'.

These special factors or personality tendencies we have listed and discussed, emphasizing the factors conducive to a unique type of obsessional defence which, when carried to extremes, produces a genuine temporary mindlessness by dismantling the perceptual apparatus. This we suggest is done by the suspension of the function of attention and we have put forward some suggestions about the quality of object required to counter or forestall this dismantling tendency.

SECTION B

CLINICAL FINDINGS

Introduction to clinical findings

The main body of the book now follows, and is composed of the individual clinical reports by the various therapists of the research group. In addition there is a chapter by the editor (D.M.) relevant to the mutism of autistic children but drawing its clinical material from the psychoanalytical treatment of schizophrenic and manic-depressive patients in late adolescence. No effort has been made to restrict the individual authors within an overall framework of exposition, and for this reason a certain amount of overlap will appear in the descriptions of the children and their analytic material. But in a way this is all to the good, for it not only enriches the concepts by multiplying the illustrations with small variations, but also serves to bind together the group of children being described. It will be seen that we have been at no pains to establish the diagnosis of Early Infantile Autism by the usual psychiatric nosological canons, but have rather left this issue to sort itself out descriptively. In the long run we ourselves found the homogeneity of the material, the evolution of the transference and the revelation of central conflicts, to be both surprising and convincing in relation to our earlier doubts and debates.

It will also appear that the order of presentation has sorted itself out with internal logic, from the most ill child, Timmy, to the most recovered, Piffie. But the logic goes further than this. Taken in order, Timmy illustrates the illness itself; John the central conflict and mental pain by which it has been precipitated; Barry the defective structure of personality which develops in consequence; and Piffie the interferences with learning and adjustment which result. Taken separately, they are very different from one another. Timmy is like a moth who occasionally finds a flame to flutter near and hurts himself upon it; John is a sad waif hidden inside the tyrant's armour, banging his way out or in, one cannot tell; Barry is a monster of egocentricity, having found the means of penetrating and occupying his object, except that it keeps falling to pieces; Piffie is the wizard, an elfin scientist exploring and controlling the universe, the iron fist now in its velvet glove. But taken together they are one child, at different stages of recovery from the mindlessness into which they fled at infancy, to spare their objects and to evade the pain of seeing the damage which they could not repair and which they may even have caused.

CHAPTER THREE

Autism proper – Timmy

John Bremner and Donald Meltzer

T his sturdy and handsome boy came to treatment at the age of six years and nine months, and was seen five times per week for approximately four years with significant, but on the whole disappointing results. However, the process of the analysis as seen at the time and as comprehended in retrospect through comparison with other cases, has come to form the foundation of our conception of the Autistic State Proper. The difficulty of exposition is very great indeed and we therefore wish to outline the plan in advance so that it may be followed more easily.

We will present first a history composed of selected facts from his development, that is, facts selected because of their special relevance to the treatment experience. Then we will record one of the early sessions with Timmy, chosen because of its completeness in sampling the phenomena that he presented in the playroom. Upon this background of history and clinical description we will then describe in a more general way the transactions of the first three years of the treatment in order to demonstrate how the mind and body of the therapist came gradually into possession of a consortium of qualities and functions that could pull together the child's scattered mentality. Only then could a process recognizable as infantile transference evolve. Finally we will describe the transference events and their outward manifestations during a period in the fourth year centring on a most interesting lapse in Timmy's previously well-established faecal continence.

Developmental history

Timmy was the third of four children of a united couple and the only manifestly disturbed child. The parents were intelligent and well-educated upper-middle-class people, and the father's high position in an international firm required that they live abroad. The two exceptions to this were a period of prolonged convalescence for the mother when Timmy was five months old, and the first three years of his psychotherapy.

The first five months of his life were a delight to his mother and breast-feeding was a great success, supplemented by bottles only during a holiday journey in the third month, which the baby tolerated well. His entire care was in the mother's hands despite the presence of a nanny, until the illness which required mother's hospitalization and sudden weaning of the baby at five months. Perhaps 'sudden' is too strong a term, for in the premonitory two weeks of the illness increasing supplementation by bottle and increasing activity by the nanny were necessary.

The absolute separation from the mother was only a few weeks and no noticeable setback in Timmy's development declared itself. By eleven months he was standing well, could say 'mummy,' and 'daddy' quite distinctly, was alert and cheerful. On his first birthday he walked free. But the relationship between mother and child had not recovered, on either side, as his care slipped imperceptibly more and more to the devoted nanny. When she had to return to her native country one month after this triumph of walking alone, Timmy was inconsolable, alternately crying and raging, rejecting mother except for being read to. Night-time grieving went on for many months during the family's return abroad despite Timmy's friendly acceptance of a new nanny who gently toilet-trained him over the next year. In this second year Timmy was cheerful and friendly, progressed in his speech and was noticeably prone to make people laugh. Mother became pregnant with Bobby shortly before Timmy was due to go to hospital for repair of his small umbilical hernia, at two years one month. This proved a thoroughly traumatic affair from which the father dates the child's deterioration, although its manifestations were only made apparent after the birth of Bobby. In retrospect it could be seen that the eight months separating these two events were not ones of much progress in speech; he seemed to become somewhat more of a spectator than participant in family life. Perhaps his continence lapsed a bit; perhaps certain tic-like repetitions appeared in his speech. The one indubitable worry was that he ran away from home for the first time when mother was nearing term in her pregnancy.

But the sequellae to the birth of Bobby were unmistakable and rather frightening. Bobby seemed quite invisible and inaudible to Timmy; his speech, which had already been composed of clearly delineated English and French, dried up; a nursery school attempt failed as did an attempt at psychotherapy. He seemed to need either mother or nanny present continually, had unexplained outbreaks of crying or rage, was banging his head against the wall and rushing aimlessly about biting his fist when upset. His only new accomplishment was to learn to ride a bicycle, but because of his tendency to ride off, mother had to rope him to herself when taking him to the park. When his nanny left he accepted a new one but the grieving returned and his behaviour became 'more clearly destructive towards the mother's possessions, especially the flowers in her garden. At times he would just stay in bed and refuse to eat, while giving himself lots of little drinks. He could not bear to be praised, tore paper a lot and quickly destroyed anything he made in plasticine or sand.

Timmy was six years nine months when the family decided to try a second psychotherapeutic effort, which they then supported very well for four years in the face of great difficulty and some degree of disappointment. To supplement this historical data, we wish now to add a description of an early session of the analysis. We will mark the places at which some descriptive or interpretive activity was undertaken by the therapist with an asterisk (*) but not give its content. In general at this time the therapist, of course, comprehended nothing very specific and confined himself fairly largely to a sort of running commentary in which the child's activities and emotions were described in terms of the most infantile type of relationships and objects, including any indication of transference.

Fifteenth session: Monday

'Timmy comes in with a blue raincoat and looks dark and determined. He rushes to the window (which overlooks a charming garden) and shakes his fist. I offer to take his coat and he allows this but immediately rushes about the room in a wild way shaking his fist at the chairs, the light, and perhaps the flowers in the garden. Timmy then empties the bag of plasticine which he has taken from the box of toys, chews some and spits it out all over the room in a seemingly random way. He goes to the sink, takes the mug, which he first bites, then fills, sips and spits on the window ledge, also pouring the remains in the corner of the ledge. (*) After about fifteen minutes of rushing about he comes to the corner where I am sitting, pours out the plasticine and stuffs some in his mouth. Now Timmy commences a complicated process of dropping bits from his mouth onto me. (*) He laughs and leans against my leg and puts bits of plasticine on my forehead. (*) Timmy goes away to the window and into thought, singing to himself and eating bits of plasticine. (*) He comes back to me, leans and sucks his thumb sadly. (*) He returns to the box, takes out a little plastic pipe, bites it. (*) He drops it and takes some plasticine over to the couch which is near my chair, reaching for my hands to pick him up, indicating by body movement something like a desire to be swung round. (*) When I say it is time to stop he seems delighted, rushes from the room and begins to suck his thumb as soon as he is through the door.

'Such a behavioural description might fit any small psychotic child. To the outline the colouring must be added to capture its true quality. At no time does Timmy appear to be listening or taking any cognizance of me that is distinguishable from his relation to the equipment of the room or the items of the garden. He makes various noises that have a vague emotive quality but no resemblance to speech. When he laughs as if at my interpretation it has no such quality but is delayed and internal. Even his terminal behaviour is not to be distinguished as a response to my saying it is time, but is the same as other times when he will suddenly dash laughing from the room in response to inner prompting. Clearly the hands are to lift him, the coat flies from him, my leg is a surface to lean against. I do not feel ignored; I feel non-existent. I am not hurt or pleased, only somehow deeply saddened by the spectacle of his incomprehensible behaviour. It tires me; I am relieved when he is gone and have to struggle to recall and record the session, knowing that if I delay it will slip through the interstices of my memory, leaving only an inchoate sadness.'

The first three years of treatment

We wish in this section to try to pull together the mass of phenomena that Timmy presented in the playroom, into some sort of order so that the evolution of a transference process can become apparent. But we also wish to do this in a descriptive way that is as free as possible from the jargon of the particular theoretical framework within which the interpretive work was being done. The general trend of Timmy's behaviour and feeling appeared to us to fall into two categories initially, later a third and gradually a fourth. The first two of these, his sensual relation to objects and his bodily relation to space, were at first so primitive and fragmented that only very gradually did the third dimension, his relation to time, and the fourth, his phantasy relation to objects, make their appearance. We came gradually to construe that this primitiveness of sensual relation to objects and bodily relation to space were the essential properties of the Autism Proper, from which he could later emerge for longer and longer periods in order to take up an existence in time and a relation to phantasy objects.

The Autism Proper appeared to be composed of a galaxy of items in random relation to one another. The fifteenth session shows something of this but we must give a more complete description. Timmy's autistic behaviour seemed to us to be composed of sensual events which had at best a most tenuous continuity. From the very beginning he took a sensuous interest in certain items – perhaps 'interest' is too complex a term. For the four years of the treatment these items and his mode of contact with them remained unchanged. He tended to suck the window latch, bite the little calf, suck the cow, drink from and spit into the mug, shake his fist at the garden, flowers, birds or children in neighbouring gardens, to mutter and shake his fingers, hand in mouth, at the dots and lines of the lino, lean against the couch or therapist's leg, listen to distant sounds of airplanes, lick the glass of the window, smell the plasticine or seat, stroke the analyst's face, masturbate against the couch or the therapist's knee, bite the plastic pipe.

From this dazzling display we came to believe that in the Autistic State Proper, a kind of mindlessness existed in which his sensory equipment was dismantled from a united or consensual mode of functioning. It appeared that each modality tended to seek out a separate item of the environment to make contact with, and that the motor behaviour associated with it was of the most rudimentary, mechanical, phantasy-free type, having neither sources in previous items nor consequences for subsequent ones. Insofar as they seemed to be the debris of decomposed phantasies and object relationships, the interpretive activity of the therapist was aimed at identifying the fragmented image, much as an archaeologist will reconstruct a vase from the debris of a midden. This is, in a sense, very different from the ordinary analytic practice of reconstructing the unconscious phantasy from its conscious derivatives. This would correspond to the archaeologists' reconstruction of a culture from the artifacts, involving an elevation of interpretation to a higher level of abstraction. In that sense the therapist's interpretations of the Autistic Phenomena Proper could hardly be called psychoanalytic, as they did not undertake to discern the anxieties and defences, the meta-psychology, that is, but only to bring together the fragments of dismantled experience. We do not mean to say that this is what he set out to do. It is all hindsight; this is what he seems to have found himself doing in fact, *faute de mieux*.

Accompanying this dismantled sensual relation to objects Timmy presented what seemed to be a near total confusion regarding the geography of his environment when in the Autistic State Proper. He would tend to dive into the room, to push his head against the glass of the garden door. He could appear to be triumphant over the birds in the garden one moment and jealously threatening them the next. Equally he could dive onto the couch or push his head into the cushions; or just as well he could dive onto the therapist or push his head into his abdomen. Timmy might look intently out of the window and a moment later look equally intently into the therapist's mouth or ear or eye. His attempts to run out of the room could not be distinguished from running into it — into the garden, into the couch, into the therapist's arms. Spitting out of his mouth, into the room, into the mug, out of a hiding place seemed either so indistinguishable or the orientation of inside and outside so quickly reversible as to be inconsequential. A sound could seem to invade his space as concretely as the sight of a workman in the garden.

From these aspects of Timmy's behaviour, coupled with the degree of his surface contact with objects, we construed that his life-space was so shapeless, that his object, and probably therefore his body, was so two-dimensional that there was no hiding-place in the world of his autism and no object that could be possessed in an internal hiding-place. Indeed he never seemed to put things in or out of his pockets; things taken into mouth or hand seemed to come out again so quickly that one had the impression that they had virtually fallen through him. But this surface, two-dimensional quality of Timmy's world had a tormenting aspect that went beyond the frustration of his impulse to hide himself in an object or to hide it possessively within himself. These surfaces seemed fairly crawling with minute rivals. These were especially represented by the dots on the lino and the birds in the garden. It often seemed that he was driven from object to object, sensory modality to sensory modality, by this distressing contamination. While in the early months only a growling of impotent rage accompanied these experiences, out of his nearly absolute mutism there eventually emerged the clearly defined words 'baby' and 'Bobby', used interchangeably.

At first everything was thus contaminated. Gradually it became more localized in the vague human shapes of a colourful print of Dufy's 'Ascot' which hung on the playroom wall. By the fourth year it had begun to fasten itself on the occasional sounds of the therapist's children coming from upstairs in the house. The material we will present shortly from the fourth year was some-what precipitated by the only incident in which Timmy actually caught a glimpse of one of the therapist's little boys when leaving a session.

But just as this contamination with Bobby-babies gradually became localized, leaving a relatively untroubled space in the room, so too did the time of the analysis become divided. In the early months the only evidence of cognizance of time Timmy manifest was that the quality of his autistic behaviour was more furious after the weekend, as in the session presented (No. 15). Soon the Fridays also took on this complexion and gradually the holidays became fraught. The grieving behaviour reported in the history reappeared and reached a crescendo in the fourth year, so that at times he was inconsolable at night, wept and banged his head, once actually thrusting it through the glass of a window.

So, too, a certain progress in the compartmentalizing of his life could be traced in retrospect. It took a most interesting form which had its anlage in the earliest sessions and its most developed form in the material of the fourth year. It will be realized that in Session 15, Timmy spat and dripped water on the ledge of the window looking on the garden. He also in most sessions would run back and forth between the entrance to the playroom and the door to the garden. These two items gradually metamorphosed into 'cordonning' and 'mirror' behaviour.

The cordonning came first and consisted of the use of spit, later also urine, to seal the playroom off from the garden, as if with a mine field. Once this had been established, a new form of terminal behaviour tended to appear to replace either the happy-rushing-off seen in Session 15, or the more frequent curling-up-and-refusing-to-leave. What Timmy discovered was his image in the hallway mirror, and he began to take leave of his mirror-image, often with various methods of showing his tongue.

Now all this time, the first three years of the analysis, in which transference space was being cleared in the debris of the Autistic State Proper, another development was taking place which gradually altered the aesthetic quality of the hours. From a process in which occasional items of transference could be located in the welter of autistic phenomena, something more linked together emerged. A transference process could be seen to be embedded in a matrix of autistic items. This process was a most direct one indeed and came gradually to be more and more centred on a particular object, the therapist's head, perhaps even his mind. The items of contact with the therapist's body, some of which appeared in Session 15, and had that impersonal quality which made them indistinguishable from contact with the inanimate things of the room, changed in consistent and characteristic ways. Two regions became important, the area beneath the therapist's chair and his head.

While early in the treatment Timmy characteristically took items one by one from the box of toys and then discarded them angrily at random after a cursory bite, suck or smell, this randomness altered into a fairly regular pattern of casual distribution into the corners of the room, under the couch or beneath the sink. The wastepaper basket later entered into this, but finally toys began to be dropped in the therapist's lap and eventually to be collected under his chair.

Coincident with this trend, Timmy's behaviour toward the therapist's head became increasingly personal and complicated. He looked into his orifices, stroked his checks and hair, licked him and smelled his breath. Sometimes he would try to shut his mouth with hand or elbow while he was talking. But eventually more and more he would put his ear near the therapist' s mouth and even put his own mouth close and make sucking or eating movements. But the glasses and moustache were his enemies, or at least rivals, and would be attacked in various ways. Upon this backdrop of converging attachment a drama began to take shape which we will now present in some detail: the 'squeezing material'. We intend to cull out of the autistic matrix on the one hand and the repetitiveness of the obsessionality on the other hand, a string of items that will tell the story, indicating the session number for each.

The 'squeezing' material

By this time Timmy's family had had to return abroad and he had been left in the care of the housekeeper who, along with her husband and son, somewhat older than the patient, were tenderly devoted to this charming and attractive boy. He was talking in short phrases quite a lot, English, French and Italian; and gave little difficulty in his management. During the mornings he attended a small specialized school where he was very popular, moderately socialized and somewhat constructive, but still fundamentally ineducable (Session 697). It was three days before he reacted to seeing the therapist's little boy, but when the storm broke it was a hurricane of rage and clinging, accompanied by a deterioration in his usually robust health, but a paradoxical increase in his language, including chanting 'Oh, my darling, oh, my darling' to the recognizable tune of 'Clementine' (700). Timmy's cough worsened after the therapist was obliged to cancel a session. He cried most of the night, was thought to have an earache, ate little and was kept in bed for two days. But in the ten days' holiday that followed, Timmy was well and cheerful, except that be did not defaecate for the three days before returning to the analysis (703). He was very excited before this session, repeatedly called the therapist 'naughty boy', and on leaving, when looking in the mirror, pointed to the therapist and repeated this accusation (706). The sound of hammering next door made him grin and say, 'Daddy', but (707) when it was repeated he buried his head in the therapist's chest and sobbed, putting his mouth close to the therapist's when he talked (710). He now seemed a bit frightened of the birds in the garden, tending to cover his mouth when they flew past. In this context the first incident of squeezing occurred. It consisted of standing balanced on one leg and bearing down, becoming quite red in the face. He was constipated, seemed often to have pains in his tummy (714). Timmy seemed also more coldly destructive at times now, treading on the little plastic calf saying 'kill, kill' and seemed to mean it. When (715) he reached into the box and pulled out the calf, he burst into tears and was inconsolable until he found the cow where he had in fact discarded it under the therapist's chair (716). Now to this drama of squeezing, constipation and violence a kind of blowing was added, which also involved blowing into the mouth of the therapist. Soon after (721) he was ill with fever and a gastric flu which brought his mother home to visit and take him away for a week's convalescence. She was delighted with Timmy's progress and felt closer to him than she ever had since he was an infant. But he did not defecate the entire week, refused all cathartics and did not pass a motion until after returning to the analysis (729). In that session he fell and hurt himself slightly, though he took it rather smilingly (733). His squeezing was now accompanied by farting, sometimes with his backside pointed at the garden, sometimes also blowing and making bubbles with his mouth (734). The following session he dropped the cow into the wastebasket, retrieved it, then began to play in a new way with the basket, rolling it, admiring his reflection in the surface, hugging it on the couch while masturbating, saying 'po-po'. After a cursory hug of the therapist's head, he returned to the wastebasket, tried to climb inside and finally lay on the floor with one leg in it, sucking his thumb.

His use of language was increasing rapidly in the sessions now. So also the quality of communication that his behaviour reflected (741). He pretended to he fighting imaginary foes, blowing, farting, spitting and shouting 'Get out' at them on the Friday. On the Monday (747) he dropped a ball of faeces from his trousers while squeezing, but immediately rolled on it so that it seemed almost to disappear into his clothes. This marked the start of a long siege in the analysis which, since it begins to merge with the phenomena well known from the treatment of non-autistic and non-schizophrenic psychotic children, is not particularly germaine to our presentation. We have in a sense reached the point of onset of Timmy's autism and the point of arrest in his development. The autistic fragments that were seen in Session 15 have now come alive once more. The mindlessness of the autism is being replaced by the reinstatement of the developmental process. But Timmy is ten years old at this point, while his developmental age is about two. The appearance of the analyst's child had precipitated this dramatic repetition of Bobby's birth.

What, then, do we feel has been the accomplishment of analysis up to this point, leaving aside for a moment the attenuation of the child's recourse to autistic states? We think that he has achieved the formation of an object that has a space inside it suitable for the reception of the child's mental pain (the wastebasket and space beneath the therapist's chair). There also appears to be an object, the therapist's head, from which he can introject something comforting, perhaps even already nurturing, into his internal world. It would appear from his squeezing material and the attendant somatic disturbance that he now had an internal world from which he could banish his rivals, relegating them to the external world (the Dufy picture and the therapist's children upstairs). This localization of his rivals does seem to enable him to distinguish them from his persecutors (the hammering next door) although these are not as yet clearly distinguished from the daddy in intercourse with the mummy (his first response to the hammering). Thus the structural groundwork for personality development seems to have been laid. But it is dreadfully late and the habit of employing the autistic manoeuvre is very strong. It is clear from the sessions that in the face of mental pain he still retreats and has to be pulled together by the attractiveness of the analyst's head-breast and voice-milk.

Recapitulation

Can we now in any measure relate the findings of the analytic process to the few well-established facts of Timmy's developmental history? After such patient work and restraint of imagination, we may allow ourselves a bit of a flight of fancy. This intelligent and highly sensual baby enjoyed a very sequestered bliss in the first five months, virtually never left alone, whether it was in mother's arms, at the breast or in the care of his doting nanny. Did he phantasy that this state was the achievement of his successful faecal attacks on mother's internal babies only to discover that he had poisoned the breast? His mother's illness was a slowly commencing hepatitis and she fed Timmy for two weeks of its onset. Did the milk taste bitter? Did her yellowing complexion declare his guilt? The bottle may have brought a relief from this catastrophic guilt but it required the sacrifice of his very sensual relation to mother's body as well, only to find that the expected punishment (the umbilical surgery) eventuated nonetheless. When his mother's swelling abdomen declared the triumph of his rival, there was nothing for it but 'kill, kill' or run away in search of the nanny who had rescued him from the first debacle. This running away was beyond his physical means, so he had recourse to running away from being himself. But this required a most severe operation. How a child can find these means remains a most awesome mystery.

Discussion

The case of Timmy, perhaps because he was the most severely disordered of the children we studied, gradually became the cornerstone about which the conception of Autism and Post Autism was erected during the years of systematic review of the material in seminar. Nonetheless, we often feel that we have only stripped the surface richness from the material, as each rewriting has shown. Like some of the cave walls of the Dordogne where the animals have been inscribed rather than painted, every shift of the beam of light brings a new animal to view from the welter of scribble. Some of the interesting questions raised by Timmy's behaviour will find an even richer or more pointed exposition in other children's material. For instance, it will be seen that John's mental state at the onset of his treatment more or less takes off where Timmy has reached after four years. The same will be seen in regard to Barry and then to Piffie. For this reason they have arranged themselves in a linear way and could virtu- ally be strung together to make the story of one child and one reasonably complete and successful analysis. Timmy does truly demonstrate most clearly the operation of the autistic manoeu- vre and its juxtaposition to phantasy and object relations. John does really show the part played by the catastrophic depressive pain impinging on a naked organism. Barry does really show step by step the process of building an object with an internal space and a self with an internal world. Piffie does really demonstrate in brilliant detail the obsessional mechanisms which created the autism, applied in a constructive way to modulate the pain of the developmental process and how they do also interfere with learning. But all four of the children also do demonstrate all of the aspects in varying degrees.

So we will restrict ourselves here to the discussion of those aspects of the experience with Timmy which will not find better illustration elsewhere.

The first question that arises is the relation of the autistic manoeuvre to suicide. Are we dealing with the ultimate example of what Melanie Klein, referring to children's accidents, called 'suicide attempts with as yet insufficient means'? Can we see Captain Oates walking off into the ice-field in Timmy's first wandering away from home? This idea is in no way in compatible with the thought that he was going to search for his first nanny and would seem to characterize depressive suicide of the non-violent, not self-mutilating sort. It seems to us a cogent view of the Autistic State Proper that it truly, more than any other form of mental derangement, would deserve the appellation of 'losing one's mind'. The fact that it seems so momentarily reversible appears to us a most wonderful invention of non-violence. But this leads on to the next question.

Is our view of autism as a total mental state rather than a split one tenable? On what evidence do we base this conclusion that the reversibility is something fundamentally different from the rapid shifting of states of mind seen where splitting is very severe and where the sense of identity has not been firmly anchored, as in most non-schizophrenic psychotics, or in adolescents? We did in fact start out with the assumption that we were witnessing the operation of splitting processes and only after some years came to hold this different view. This, we think, is not surprising, for the evidence is in fact rather retrospective of necessity. If we compare the Timmy of the 'squeezing' material with the child of Session 15 we see that nothing has changed other than the architecture. All the building materials were present at the very start, but only after four years is a structure of a personality with internal and external objects visible. Truly even after such efforts Timmy is no better off than the first little pig in his house of straw, but one can see the possibility of a house of sticks and eventually one of bricks that will not be blown down by every passing wolf of mental pain.

This implies that we feel that the processes that we have studied in these children are either purely pathological and play no part in ordinary developmental history, or else that they are so early as to be proximal in developmental time to the point where schizoid mechanisms can be brought into operation. Work with other types of patients of very varying severity of illness but where fragility of the organization of the ego is a central problem would seem to suggest the latter. The pioneer work in this area is that of Mrs Esther Bick on the psychic function of the skin, which serves to give clinical substance to Wilfred Bion's exposition of the concept of container-and-contained in mental life.

This attitude seems further strengthened by the evidence that the dismantling type of primitive obsessional mechanism plays a role in the formation of the fetish, as described by one of the authors (D.M.) These theoretical problems will be discussed further in the various chapters of Section C.

We may shift our angle a little and look at this developmental process from a slightly different point of view. What we would like to consider here is the possible part played by the intensity of sensation, and the single mode of sensory perception in Timmy's autism.

In the previous chapter mention was made of 'triumphant joyous possession of the maternal object' as a feature common to all these children. It was certainly present in Timmy but in a different way from the way it appeared in Barry and Piffie and perhaps in a slightly different way from the way it appeared in John to whom Timmy was most akin. The difference appears to lie in the degree of structure of Timmy's mind and in its nature.

To understand this we must look at the terms more closely. If we look at the term 'triumph' we see that it implies someone possessing some thing, or state, which he is aware some rival does not possess. The fact that one may triumph in achievement does not really exclude the notion of a rival, for the difficulty tends to be personified as the rival over whom one triumphs. To experience triumph the concept of rival must exist in some form however dim within the mind. For Timmy it is very possible that this concept existed more in a concrete form within his own body, than in any way as a developed object within his own mind, though it certainly invaded his mind, and was there developed enough to be projected in a recognizable way, though more often than not into the oddest forms such as any small object which moved, or into dots and marks on the floor. The fact that he called these Bobby/baby does show he had a mind capable of forming and containing a mental construct, but the impression we had was that both were vestigial.

The other term we would like to consider is 'possession'. 'Possession' denotes a relationship, and consciousness of it implies an awareness at least of partial identity, some awareness of the nature of the linking quality of possession, as the link between this identity and the object possessed, and some awareness of differentiation of the object from the identity and from its surroundings. These are extremely complex mental processes requiring a structured mind, and this Timmy did not seem to possess.

It was this sort of mental process which Timmy was rarely able to achieve except in a very rudimentary way. We used the word 'possessiveness' in his case, to try ourselves to understand and to give meaning to his behaviour. But for the most part this was too sophisticated a term, certainly in the first half of his treatment. He was perhaps greedy and hungry for a certain quality of sensation rather than for a maternal object.

To any mental counterpart of such an object the sensory quality often seemed only loosely attached; for we saw time after time how he would turn to any external object, even if these objects were as different themselves as a toy soldier, the corner of a table, or the surface of a piece of polished wood, provided he could suck it, lick it or stroke it. It was as if the universe contained innumerable breasts, or rather part-breasts, and that when one was lost there was always another to be found which would do just as well. This was possible because he related to it only in terms of one sensory mode. We shall see later that John too relied on a single sense datum in reality testing.

Even when Timmy was triumphant, it was rather that a part of Timmy possessed part of a maternal object from which very temporarily contaminating rivals had been excluded. The extent to which such an idea had in any way been meaningfully articulated in Timmy's mind was impossible to say. We would think hardly at all. The quality of depth in any mental process appeared to be very shallow and the process seemed to be concerned chiefly with an emotion or feeling. For him possession was rather joyous uninterfered-with contact, a sensory experience with a certain emotional quality, which may well have left no room for awareness other than of itself; from which rivals were not so much excluded as non-existent, until the awareness of the feeling either faded or changed. At this point either rivals would at once appear, to whom the loss would be attributed, or he would collapse and be overcome by an enormous wave of depressive anxiety, terminating in manic behaviour.

It was possible to see a rudimentary splitting at the moment of frustration, an attempt to expel the contaminated breast and his rivals, and an attempt to retain the good breast inside him, which did indeed give fleeting meaning to Timmy of his experience. Usually, however, this was accompanied by such rage that one could well imagine that his awareness of fury was so total as to preclude establishment of the other half of the split, that is any concept of a good inner object. Indeed, how dependent the maintenance of this inner object was upon actual sensory experience of contact, was shown by the fact that, in these states, Timmy invariably put one thumb right into his mouth, sucking it and holding it with his teeth, whilst furiously shaking his fist with the other hand at his rivals represented by dots or marks.

On the other hand, the intensity of his grief, if that were the outcome, was such as totally overwhelmed himself and his object, leaving no room for the reinstatement of the object internally, nor any place for it externally, for all his universe was grief. It was as if all good had vanished into nothingness, much as we are told may happen in the latest horrifying theory concerning the black holes in space, in which a star or even a galaxy can apparently pass out of the universe to unthinkable nowhere. Mourning, both for this reason and because he had not developed any structure within his mind of a containing place, could not therefore take place. Had he been more able to mourn he might have turned his mind from the intensity of the pain of his loss, to the memory of the good qualities of the object, and so reinstated it within him. His good object was therefore irretrievable and beyond internal symbolic recall, though not beyond the reinstatement implied in recognition. This utter loss could only intensify his grief and despair. With no other resources open to him his only recourse now was to manic omnipotent denial, frequently accompanied by the projection of rage and despair and a restless searching, until another concrete object was found to suck, to stroke, to look at or feel.

In Timmy's largely two-dimensional world there were objects affording contact to be found, and we are not saying that when he was mindless he had no memory at all, particularly of recognition or sensation, but rather that his memory appeared to approximate more towards what we might call the computer type of memory, recognition by means of sensory pattern. Even worms for instance may be taught to recognize the right path through a maze. Therefore though he had only a minimal good object inside his mind, he could get in touch with it again such as it was, since any external object, which had one of the requisite maternal qualities might have the capacity to provide a sensory awareness in some matching way. It just had to be suckable, or have a particular tactile quality, or provide some other sensation of this order.

We see, therefore, at this point a child who, because he has such a strong tendency to rely on a single mode of sensory perception, was crippled in his capacity to form meaningful inner objects or to relate adequately to external ones, or to think. The symbols by which he could develop his mind seem to be bound physically to external objects by his need for, or use of, a single sensory mode of perception which he appears unable to link with other sensations to form a meaningful whole. His behaviour emotionally and physically is chaotic and repetitive, while his memory appears to function almost totally by a very narrow recognition, rather than by symbolic recall, and to be almost exclusively concerned with his relationships to components of the breast and to a narrow field of relationships to his rivals for them.

Now let us look at Timmy at a later stage in his treatment where we see him in the playroom enacting a scene at the breast. It was not until the later years of his analysis that Timmy showed clearly that he was experiencing a number of sensations simultaneously. For instance in one session he gazed at the clouds and the blue sky, while sucking the knob of the window catch, and sometimes licking the glass. At the same time one hand could be outstretched and the tips of his fingers gently stroking the smooth paint of the wooden frame of the window, while simultaneously giving the impression of listening intently to the therapist's voice. He then got down and turned to the therapist, leaning against him, gazing into his eyes through his glasses, licking them, and then, with his mouth close to his, made eating motions with his lips as the therapist talked, while stroking his cheek and fondling his ear. Suddenly the peaceful scene broke down and Timmy thrust his thumb in his mouth and shook his fist at the pattern of small marks on the leather of the therapist's shoes. These had in previous sessions been identified with Bobby-babies.

The picture that we are seeing now is a very different one, but can we be certain that what we are seeing is a baby Timmy at the breast, rather than, say, a number of baby Timmies each with his own piece of breast? The transference is to an object not in any way closely related in itself, but widely scattered in space among the sensory perceptions of which only some come from the living source. The parts are related by being simultaneously experienced, but in each case, save perhaps in that of the voice, an enormous number of relevant qualities are being ignored to select the relevant one. The fact that he can make such skilful use of such widely disparate material tends to convince us that he actually has in mind some related idea, by which he holds the parts together. But it is only loosely held, even if with great longing, and it is not by any means complete. In particular it lacks the organizing visual quality. It has little quality of depth or flexibility, and is very concretely enacted. There is no doubt that the idea was in Timmy's mind and imposed upon the external material, but it still seems, at least partially, under the influence of single sensory perception, e.g. smoothness of the painted surface to stand for mother's skin, ignoring hardness or shape or form or temperature.

When Timmy turned to the therapist's head as a breast, we have the impression that his experience in the transference has become more focused and more vivid for him, though still very concrete. In the period of time between leaving the window and coming to the therapist, he had however relinquished the physical sensations of sucking, licking and stroking, while retaining those belonging to sight and hearing, for he looked directly at the therapist while approaching him. For this short period of time, the sensations relinquished must have been fused in some meaningful way and been associated with the sight and sound of an interrelated external object.

Finally it breaks down under the threat of rival babies, but there had been no cry of a child, no noise had invaded the consulting room, no bird flown past the window, and the therapist had not altered or stopped talking. It was almost certain that the stimulus had come from within Timmy.

Up to this point we have chiefly been considering the part which may be played by single sensations in the mode of perception, while the part played by the intensity of the sensory perception has largely been implicit. We wonder whether it may not play quite a large part.

We know that very intense sensations can interfere with and even preclude normal mental functioning. Intense pain, intense light, extremely penetrating noise, even intense pleasure can so fill the mind as to leave room for nothing else; a single strong emotion unmodified by others can have the same effect, and while not claiming that Timmy's sensory awareness was of that order, we may legitimately wonder whether it did not tend in that direction.

We may wonder whether the intensity of the original sensual experience at the breast, the delight of the mother's silkiness of skin against his cheek, the smoothness of the milk in his mouth, its delicious taste on his tongue, the exquisiteness of her scent in feeding, were not each of such ravishing pleasure to this very sensual baby, that each in itself by its very strength, made it difficult for him to pull these pieces together into a whole in the first place.

We may wonder too if such intensity of sensuality might not have been enhanced by the mother identifying herself with the baby in such a way that she experienced the baby's pleasure as her own, in order to ward off depressive anxiety, but in so doing colluded with the baby, leading to an increase in his sensuality, rather than a containment of him inside her mind in introjective identification.

If the intensity of sensory awareness did play a large part, it would tend towards a single form of sensory perception, since whichever sensation was most intense would tend to crowd out other sensations simultaneously received. This could interfere with the primitive but immensely important mental function of linking by association, making it difficult to form a consensual and coherent whole maternal object, the breast. If that were the case, such an object would be fragile and likely to fall to pieces into its constituent parts, as would the mind of the baby, neither being able to contain the other, and so would bring his mental development to a halt. This idea, akin to a concept of a sensual trauma, (colour-shock in the Rorschach?) is suggested as an extension of the descriptive term 'sensuous'.

In such a chain of events greed and jealousy would play an important role, and both were marked features in Timmy. Greed would strengthen the tendency to get the utmost from each sensation and thus increase its intensity, but in so doing defeat its aim, for habituation would the sooner set in. When it did, jealousy would be provoked. As the intensity of the pleasurable awareness faded, Timmy would become gradually aware of either other babies, or another baby Timmy, enjoying another delicious sensation. Greed would heighten his jealousy and the discordant feeling would bring about a chaotic breakdown in his relationship to the breast.

Something of this nature could have been what happened in the breakdown of his relationship to the therapist's head, representing the breast. In this state Timmy would then be not unlike a man passionately fond of music, who, when he went to listen to a rich and many-themed symphony, after a little while found himself only able to hear one instrument, and was therefore convinced that his neighbour was stealing the symphony from him.

CHAPTER FOUR

Primal depression in autism – John

Isca Wittenberg

I should like to portray some of the experiences I had with John in the course of his first year of analytic treatment with me. Much of the time, these experiences were so painful for one or both of us, that it requires considerable effort to face the task of reliving them again in one's mind. I shall describe in detail some of the sequences of play and behaviour in the hope that it will allow the reader to draw his own conclusions about the nature of John's relationships. I have in most instances not quoted the interpretations I gave, but indicated in my comments on the session how I understood what was going on. I shall want to pose many questions and only tentatively suggest some causes for John's liability to lose himself in a state of mindlessness or alternatively to collapse into a particular kind of catastrophic depression. While the unrelenting projection of despair made this child at times difficult to bear, John's passionate nature, his capacity for tenderness, his vulnerability to depressive pain, and his appeal for help evoked great affection and concern in me.

It will be seen that the material is understood against a background of theory derived from Melanie Klein's work. The need for the mother to hold the projected pain of the infantile psyche, as stressed by W. R. Bion, views the mother as container, and thus links with Esther Bick's work on the containing function of the skin. But I shall present the sessions and my reflections about them as free from technical terms as possible and aim to convey the impact of this child and the feelings he was able to engender in me.

A brief developmental history

John was born after a difficult and prolonged labour. His mother was unwell for about two months following the birth and John was therefore bottle-fed and partially cared for by his father. He was a strong sucker, an easy and lively baby, reaching his milestones rather late. But he was a jolly infant and the parents were not unduly worried. He adored his bottle and refused to be weaned onto the cup, so that he continued to drink from a bottle long after he had accepted solids. He did not relinquish it completely until he was three.

When John was seventeen months, mother had a kidney infection and was nursed at home for six weeks. The parents then went for a week's holiday, leaving John in the charge of grandparents whom he knew well. Nonetheless, by the time the parents returned, John was expressionless and began to push mother away. From that point he showed no affection or wish to communicate; often he went to play by himself in a darkened room. There was a baby in the home when John was two years nine months old until he was three. He used to poke its ears and it was on the day that the baby left that John suddenly gave up the bottle and accepted a cup instead. He still continued to drink excessively, particularly at breakfast time.

The parents became increasingly worried about John and repeatedly sought professional advice. When John was three and a half, and with great doubts about its effectiveness, they decided on psychoanalytic treatment. At the time of referral, he had a tendency to crawl all over father's body, seemed to enjoy music and was generally hyper-active. He had ripped out every plant in the garden, picked bark off trees, torn the wallpaper off his bedroom and rocked his bed so violently that he had twice broken it. In desperation the parents strapped the child in bed until he fell asleep. He tended to attack other children by scratching their faces. At three and a half years of age he still wore nappies, having acquired neither bowel nor bladder control. His speech was limited to the naming of about fifteen objects, yet he remembered places and people over a considerable time-interval. He was fascinated by aeroplanes and was said to have been so since the age of six months.

The beginning of treatment

First session: the meteor

John emerged from mother's and the au-pair girl's hands looking sombre and determined. He was a good-looking child, sturdy and well-developed with a springy gait and fast, well co-ordinated movements. He did not look at me and offered no resistance when I took his hand and led him up the stairs. He grinned briefly at the flowers on the landing. The large teddy-bear which mother had handed him was dropped as soon as we reached the consulting-room. He picked out a small aeroplane from amongst a number of small toys spread out on the table, pushed its nose into his mouth, made it swoop through the air, then put it back in his mouth. When I began to speak, he inserted it deeper. Then he swooped on a plastic cup, dropped it, saying 'mooss' in a gruff voice, leaned against my legs, took hold of the top of my ear and twisted it. He took a brown cushion from a chair, smelled it, sat on the floor pulling at. the threads of the cover with great effort and 'eh' 'ah' noises until he had managed to tear a slit in it. He pulled out some stuffing and then pushed himself between my legs and onto my lap. He arranged my arms so that they encircled his waist and presently arched his back, went rigid and thrust himself backward. I found myself holding onto him tightly to stop him falling. He laughed when I pulled him upright and made this into a kind of game. At one point I thought I heard him mumble 'roses roses', which brought to my mind the nursery rhyme and actions which usually accompany 'ringa ringa roses, a pocket full of posies, tissue, tissue, we all fall down'. At the sound of a distant aeroplane, he quickly pushed himself off my lap, listened, looked out of the window, then into the rear window of a green toy car, smelled the brown cushion, banged it onto my lap and jumped on to it with his bottom. He turned the brooch I was wearing to examine its back, then he rushed off to the couch with teddy but returned to pull me by the hand, pushed me to sit down on the couch and lay down on his stomach, curled round my body, sucking and biting into the couch cover. Suddenly, he lunged forward, diving headfirst off the end of the couch. When I held onto him and pulled him back, he laughed and turned this into a game. Twice I let him go and he landed on his head and subsequently sucked his forearm, looking lost and forlorn. When I told John that it was time to go home but I would see him tomorrow, he stood leaning against my legs. I took him by the hand but he appeared limp and unable to walk, so I carried him downstairs. He walked off between Mother and the au-pair girl, holding their hands without looking back.

Comment. It is difficult to convey the impact which John made on me, a mixture of feeling desired, invaded, and needed all at once. Similarly it is hard to transmit the forcefulness and passion with which John took possession of me; the way he grabbed the aeroplane, tore at the threads, plucked the stuffing, forced my legs to receive him, rocked, buried his teeth in the couch, thrust himself backwards. I felt bewildered and intruded upon by his ear-pulling tyranny. But there was a power he exerted over me far more compelling than having to be the slave of his desires – the power he exerted by his appeal for help and the readiness of his suicidal impulses. John's behaviour seemed designed to show me that he needed to insert a part of me deep inside his mouth like the plane-nose, encircle and envelop it like the teat his mother reports he had so tenaciously held on to. Similarly he needed to be held, enveloped by my lap and arms. He conveyed that the alternative was to fall off like the roses; he embedded himself in my lap with the speed and force of a meteor and I felt impelled to hold onto him lest he hurl himself further into space and be lost. His limpness at the end of the session strongly suggested that it was a catastrophe to be separated – dropped, something beyond hopelessness, more a despairing apathy, cut off from life itself. He came 'to life' again when mother and the girl took his hands and seemed to need this physical handing-over to avoid the feeling of a gap.

Although I made verbal comments in line with these impressions in very simple language, I felt that the pertinent communication was on a non-verbal level. While normally I would discourage any physical contact, John not only demanded it but seemed to express an imperative need for it. I did not feel that I was dealing with a three-year-old child but with a young infant, terrified of falling into an abyss.

Second session: the tip-up lorry

John looked more lively and came upstairs with an eager step. He excitedly smelled the brown cushion and me, went once round my chair, stood by my side, looked at my face and, laughing, jumped up and down in a bouncy way. He noticed a red ball in a bowl, picked it up and threw it away. He ran off with the aeroplane, making humming noises, touched his penis briefly and lay on the couch rocking and laughing. At the sound of an aeroplane he jumped up, slapped my arm, saying 'daddy' and smelled my legs. He took the aeroplane and green car to the couch and held the plane's nose to the back of the car, looked into its rear window, then bounced up and down on his knees. He had a laughing babbling 'conversation' with the car, then suddenly arched his back and thrust his head over the end of the couch. He came and pulled me by the ear, pushed me to sit down by the couch, and lay on his back across my lap; then he pushed the top of the tip-up lorry up and down, giving me the occasional hard slap on the back. This went on for a while, with John straining and farting. Suddenly the tip-up lorry dropped behind the couch, out of sight. John looked forlorn, held onto my ear-lobe, pulling hard at it, then held up his arms to be lifted onto my lap and sat huddled against my chest. Gradually he came to lie back in my arms, still holding on tightly to my ear-lobe, and looked intently into my eyes. Then he got up, took a ball in each hand, licking one and biting the other several times. He was reluctant to let go of them at the end of the session and gave them each a hard farewell bite.

Comment. I shall select only a few items from this very rich material. Firstly, one is struck by the great emphasis on smell, as a way of identifying objects; perhaps John had an illusion that his flatus created a barrier, a circle round me like his curled body the day before. At first indeed he behaved as if I were the red ball-breast that had been unfaithful with the daddy and must either be thrown away or forcefully repossessed. My unfaithfulness appears to have been experienced only when the sound of the aeroplane entered his consciousness. His hitting me while saying 'daddy' suggests that the aeroplane was not felt to be outside and at a distance but had intruded into John's life-space, competing with him for occupation of my room and body. For a few minutes he seemed to feel that he could be inside and participating in the mummy-daddy intercourse relationship, but his slapping and farting betrayed his jealousy. Thus John at the outset, like Timmy after four years of treatment, does not differentiate clearly between outside the room and inside the room, inside or outside my body – or alternatively his eyes have the ability to reverse the perspective (Bion) in a moment (or his fingers to turn the skin back when he twisted my ear-lobe or brooch), so that inside and outside seem to change places instantly. They become reversed as if he had gone through a revolving door. Nor is his body much differentiated from mine: 'daddy', can apparently be as easily slapped out of my back as tipped out of his own bottom. However, there seems to be a danger point where, in the process of throwing out 'daddy', he might lose 'mummy' too, or John himself might fall overboard as if from a tip-up lorry. At that moment he felt lost and forlorn and held on tightly to my ear-lobe, my arms and eyes. His capacity for gratitude when I picked him up, was indicated by his licking one ball and separating-off his anger onto the other: but such splitting quickly broke down in the face of the inevitable separation at the end of the session. Indeed I was not again to have such close contact with him for some time.

The next four and a half weeks: thrown away on the shores of lostness

In the third session John played with the aeroplane and tip-up lorry but very soon dropped both behind the couch. He began plucking different coloured pieces of plasticine into small fragments and said 'flower' in a deep, husky voice. He brought the bits to me and made it clear that I was to roll them together into a ball-shape. When I had done so, he got very excited, skipped to the couch and chewed large chunks from the plasticine ball. He screamed at the end of this session and pulled hard at the other children's drawers.

After the first weekend, he banged his head into the chest of drawers, flung the rubber ball into the fire saying 'gone', dropped the plastic cups onto the floor and threw away the plasticine ball saying 'not for eating'. Then he sat scraping plasticine off the sole of his shoe and ate that! Everything good had 'gone', as I had in the weekend. Did he feel that I had flung him away carelessly, leaving him only the plasticine-faecal food on his shoe ? Was his despair and rage compounded by jealousy of these flower-children who were held and fed in his stead? Why was the plasticine ball 'not for eating,? To spare it from his sharp teeth? I was probably blamed for allowing John and his objects to fall to bits.

For the next four weeks I saw a child in front of me whose eyes had become lifeless, who darted from one activity to another, and although his body continued to move with forcefulness, yet all his activities seemed disjointed. How can one describe purposeful aimlessness? Even in the telling it assumes an ordering of events which is alien to it. John licked, bit, discarded toys, made shape-less sounds, leant against my legs, plucked plasticine into chunks, twisted tiny twigs which he flung over his shoulder, rushed to and fro, trod on some bits, sat on others as if by accident and stamped his feet on the stairs afterwards saying 'down down' in a voice that lost strength with every descending step. From having commenced the therapy much like Timmy in his fourth year of treatment, John now behaved like the Timmy of the fifteenth session.

Only gradually did some patterns emerge after great effort on my part to identify some of the fragments of his behaviour; or perhaps it was less what I said than the presence of my voice which pulled him back into my orbit. Thus, the smelling of the stairs on the way up began to emerge and establish itself as a way of testing whether any other feet had been up since he stamped his plasticine smells onto them. Flinging the plasticine all over my room became a way of mapping out his territory and warding off his rivals. It also became clear that making my hands roll the plasticine changed it; it became a large, long sausage which he dangled in front of his mouth in a tantalizing way.

Plasticine was not the only thing he pulled apart. He arrived each morning trailing a plant which he would skilfully pluck to pieces, leaving a trail of flower-heads and leaf-flesh on the stairs as well as in the room. He stripped the plant of its foliage until only a skeleton remained, dangled this upside-down and pushed it up and down on the floor. The shape of the remaining structure would sometimes be like that of an umbrella with the spikes turned inside-out.

There was one feature which remained constant throughout: his uncanny awareness of approaching aeroplanes. His ears detected them long before mine did. He would immediately stop whatever he was doing, pull me to the window, and hold up his arms to be lifted up onto the windowsill. As soon as the plane came into sight or could be heard booming above he would hold tightly onto my earlobe, bury his head in my shoulder and then suck his forearm. Sometimes a bird came within his field of vision and when he saw it in flight, he pressed his back against my chest and stood motionless, gazing at the birds and the flowers in the garden below. He looked infinitely forlorn at those times, as if the world beyond the glass held everything from which he was hopelessly excluded. This quiet spell would be broken suddenly by his looking into my eyes, poking into my ears, slapping my shoulder fiercely and banging his head into mine. It seems that my eyes were as transparent as the windowpane and that my inside could also be looked into. It was absolutely equated with the garden where he spied the rival bird- and flower-babies, but at the same time those rivals appeared to erect a hard barrier like the pane of glass, penetrable only by banging and forcing his way in. It seemed that the presence of aeroplanes, birds and flowers meant that these rivals had taken complete possession of me and shut him out ; that there was no separate life-space which he could own, no hiding-place from them: either they or he must own the totality of the mother's body. Again, how like Timmy in the fourth year of treatment was John in the fourth week.

In retrospect, the fragments of his behaviour could be conceived of as shells, each containing aspects of his relationship with me; a constant attempt to take hold of a bit of my contents, which, though momentarily attractive, was felt to be spoilt by his biting or alternatively to be ripped away by his rivals, leaving him on the shores of despair. Driven by rage and desperation, John was not only tipping out, plucking, stripping, tearing and discarding my contents (leaving me as devastated an object as his parents' garden), but throwing away his own mind alongside these objects. He looked vacant, and appeared to have scattered his thoughts and mental functions, strewn them to the wind, when I led him 'down, down', as if he could not bear the terror of being dropped. Yet, John did not want to go under; he was strap-hanging onto my ear-lobe with the grim determination of someone holding on to dear life.

The twenty-sixth session: the attractive object – the hope-breast

Just when it seemed that his fragmented play would go on endlessly, there was a dramatic change. The stimulus was a patch of sunlight on the wall of the consulting room. John noticed it as he entered on that Monday morning, the 26th session, and for the first time a frightened expression showed on his face. It lasted only an instant, to be replaced by a grin. I commented that the bright spot was like a week-end daddy-sunshine inside me. John rushed to the drawer, swooped on a bunch of pencils, swung them around inside the elastic band which held them together. He then spread them out fanwise so that the shape looked unmistakably like a bird or aeroplane. He then let each pencil fall out in turn, pulled the elastic into an oval shape and, salivating heavily, sucked it. I said he felt that daddy had filled me up with good things but that John thought he could only get to the mummy-food once he had thrown out all these daddy-pencil parts. He opened my mouth, pushed his finger inside, took it out and smelled it, made sucking movement and starting babbling. He said 'lolly-pops' as he picked up the remains of the sweet-pea plant he had brought up with him that morning, put his arms up and propelled me to the window. While standing on the windowsill, he held his penis which was in erection. He wanted me to open the window (which I refused to do) watched the trees and birds and finally let himself 'fly' joyfully into my arms.

Comment. In John's primitive world objects which have some similarity of shape or functional association, are easily inter changeable or, more correctly, are not differentiated. Thus elastic can equal mouth = breast = window which opens; white patch equals milk = saliva = words; pencils equal penises = nipples; tongue = finger = penis. In this session John seemed to me to be on the verge of holding two part-objects together in his mind: mother and father parts joined in an enriching way, a sunshine daddy making mummy's wall-skin gleam, her breasts full; colour pencils filling mummy with food and my mouth with words. Their conjunction frightens him, but it also brought hope, liberated him from the apathy induced by living in the dungeon-bottom-mummy, and made me into an exciting, bright object. The idea seemed to occur to him that he could possess himself of it in a new way; it is as if he were saying to himself, 'I'll just throw out these daddy-parts and myself become the tongue-finger-penis flying inside this mummy-therapist'. I was deeply impressed by the intelligence which this play suggested. Furthermore this leap forward when I appeared bright and full, opened up the possibility that he might find his way back to a relationship with me. It suggested that his loss of contact had been at least partially due to a fear that his throwing me away had made me be 'gone', burnt up, bitten up. Yet how threatened was this relationship by his possessiveness and fierce jealousy?

The illusion of having penetrated me and ousted 'daddy' carried over into the next few sessions. Thus, after stripping the plants each morning, he would now skip around the table and dance in circles, holding up his fingers spread out fan-wise, looking triumphantly at the easy chair in the corner, whispering provocatively, 'daddy'. As his dancing became more and more excited, so did his laughter reach a crescendo before he flung himself into my lap. His victories were short-lived, however, for the sound of an aeroplane or the sight of a bird easily destroyed the illusion, made him slap me fiercely and retreat into sadness and then to plasticine-play.

Reflections on the nature of John's relationship: occupation and pre-occupation

Reflecting on the experience of this first month of John's analysis, a number of thoughts occur to me. I always had the strong impression that it was a matter of life and death for him to gain total possession of the analyst-mother, and all that was equated with her. This really amounted to the totality that was within sight and hearing, i.e. not only my body but the garden, the sky, the room, the aeroplane, the furniture, the contents of my body. I was struck by the fact that he not only lost me when I was absent, but so easily experienced me as lost despite my physical presence. The rivals, whether aeroplanes or birds or plants, were evidently able to take me over as soon as they appeared. My contents were at one moment all his, and at the next, all theirs. Like territory continually fought over by enemy armies, the occupation by one automatically seemed to imply the driving-out of the other. Although barricades as hard as glass or the bones of my forehead were created by John's enemies, they could be spied through, holes could be poked, one could bang one's way in. Moreover, this 'mummy' appeared to be quite passive, to offer no resistance to the invasion of her territory, to its being overrun by this or that force; she gave herself over to having her boundaries violated, so that one could tear a hole into her, as into the cushion cover, pluck some of the stuffing out or pull the whole of her skin off like the flesh of plants, leaving just a skeleton or ruin for children to run in and out of. These struts transversing the empty spaces of her structural framework were elastic, like the rubber band when robbed of the pencils. The object could be pressed into any desired shape – but at a terrible price, for this shapeless mother who does not protect herself from invasion, cannot hold and protect her baby. She has no internal space defined by firm boundaries and hence offers no hiding place from rivals; she has no membrane in which to catch and envelop John securely, nor can she catch and hold the fragments of his mental experience; she provides no bedrock for the foundations of a structure of memory or continuity of experience, for links to be forged, for phantasy to grow and develop.

What kind of experience might have led to such a concept of a mother? When I think back to John's first session, his forceful entry into my lap, I find myself wondering whether this child experienced his mother as literally preoccupied. John's parents were devoted to him and gave him ample care and attention. But could an ill mother, a depressed mother, preoccupied with her own thoughts and problems, convey the impression to her baby of warm attentiveness? Such a mother may neither offer much aliveness of response nor much resistance to being poked into. Might her inaccessibility stir a very sensuous, loving baby like John to tear into her to get at her withheld contents while her fragility would cause him to spare her from his forceful attacks? And when the parents actually left him, did he feel totally expelled, forgotten, fallen out of their minds? I felt that his plasticine play, his withdrawnness and lostness, were probably repetitions of the experience of the dark room to which he often retreated after the parents' return from holiday. These are merely questions and conjectures. All I can say with conviction based on experience is that John was extremely sensitive to my states of mind, that he reacted to any lapse of attention, any illness, physical malaise or silence as if I had rejected him. Then he either withdrew or became more hyperactive, banging into objects. I learned from experience that I must not let him drop from my mind for a moment, but needed to be alert to catch his escapes into mindlessness. At such a point it was vital to keep on talking, although it might simply be a running commentary on his actions; for my alive interest and response appeared to be the psychic equivalent of holding him, and my voice the spring that pulled him together.

Second month: the 'Laby'

During the course of the second month, my mouth and abdomen became the focus of John's interest. He would frequently insert his finger into my mouth and smell it before inserting it into his mouth. His increasing vocabulary seemed to suggest that some primitive identification was taking place, through the concrete experience of taking the saliva-words out of my mouth and putting them into his own. He often sought out my lap, lay back in my arms, snuggled against my breasts. Sometimes he would then say 'laby', which I took to mean lady-with-baby. I did not feel him at that moment to be 'inside' me as an inside-baby; rather that he was telling me that we were stuck together like the words, amalgamated, skin-to-skin. The end of sessions continued to be very distressing for him. He showed this by going limp. He would then begin the following day by tearing flesh off the leaves.

Yet his demeanour in the mid-part of sessions and the mid week was now characterized by a much gentler quality. On occasion he knelt on my thighs, put his ear to my stomach as I spoke, smelled the finger he inserted in my mouth, then pulled up his vest, touched his navel and smelled his finger afterwards. A different concept of body boundaries appeared to be developing. It was at once more definite – a skin separated inside from outside, him from me, and at the same time it was soft, not hard as before. It allowed claustrums to exist and to be carefully explored: my mouth, his mouth; my stomach, his stomach. My words which were felt to rise from my stomach up to my mouth could be put into his mouth and stomach. Although smell was still the leading sensual modality, he had begun to explore the texture, warmth and depth of the various orifices. From this point onwards John became a physically vulnerable child, easily susceptible to colds and diarrhoea. This was all the more striking because he had been in robust health for several years. His vulnerability seemed to go hand in hand with his closeness to me, and his destructive attacks quickly set off somatic deterioration. How would a holiday break affect him now? It was a worrying prospect; and it seemed essential that he should have many weeks of preparation for it, to work over his feelings about the separation and loss.

Third month: preparation for holiday – 'lady gone'

It was clear that John had developed a very intense and close relationship with me and responded to my mood, my body, my voice, my words; but I was not at all sure how much he actually understood of my verbal communications. The speed and complexity with which he reacted to my explanations about the forthcoming Christmas holidays astounded me and left little doubt about his capacity to comprehend.

I had prepared a chart which showed the days of the sessions before and after the holiday as circles filled in with red, while the missing sessions were indicated by empty circles. Pointing at the appropriate circle for each day, I said 'lady here, lady here' etc. … 'lady gone, gone' etc. … 'lady back again' – lady by that time having become established as the way he and his mother referred to me. John's immediate reaction was to look out of the window and burst into peals of laughter whenever he saw a bird. I said that he was telling himself that it was those bird-children who were being left, not John, because that would be too terrible to think about. He then went to sit astride his drawer and with one clean swoop dug out all the pencils and paper and threw them onto the floor. He hit the chart, and then tried to pull me under the table where he lay down singing the tune of 'good morning, good morning, we've danced the whole night through', although the only words I could make out were 'good moling' and 'night loo'. After I interpreted that he had thrown out the pencil-daddy parts and was taking their place in my bottom and wanted me to join him in making pooh-babies, he got up, made wavy lines, filled up some circles with plasticine and then bit the lion's head right off. He went to the couch, lay with his head hanging over one end and wanting me to pull him up again.

One is reminded of similar play at the beginning of treatment. The question arises whether he felt identified with the decapitated lion-daddy, afraid of being cut off and dropped; or whether he was threatening me with suicide – decapitating himself, severing his head from his body –unless I obeyed him. When I opened the door next morning, his mother told me that John had been most impatient to come and had been banging his head against my front-door, calling 'lady lady'. He brought five sweets with him which reminded me of the five circles per week on the holiday chart. He touched and smelled my mouth, licked and sucked his sweets very carefully and slowly, putting them down for 'rests' in between, so that they in fact lasted the whole hour. All this was quite different from his usual behaviour, for he had always chewed his sweets and finished them one after the other. It became clear that these sweets were equated with time units, to be preserved in the hope that the sessions/analysis/time could equally be stretched out, be made to last for ever. For much of the time he sat on my lap, looking at the chart and repeating after me: 'lady here. . . lady gone . . . lady back again'. He rocked gently, looking increasingly sad. Then there followed a great deal of smelling of furniture, pulling threads out of the couch cover, breaking the soap and digging his nails into the pieces. But in between he came to stand quietly next to me gently licking the sweets. We see John here probably trying to split off his angry feelings onto other parts of my body/room in order to preserve the sweet/ breast.

He returned   after the weekend   with a rasping cough, plucked a big lump of plasticine to bits, and looked slyly at the 'daddy-chair, in the corner, saying 'hello fish'. He then stood on my thighs, defaecated into his pants, looked out of the window and said 'babies'. He huddled close to me, gazed into the distant horizon and said slowly and forlornly 'lady, lady, lady gone'. Then he turned to the holiday-chart and filled the blank circles with plasticine. He wiped his hand over his trouser seat, then proceeded to smell my hair, other chairs and pieces of furniture with increasing frenzy. He turned to Teddy, whom he had deposited on the table at the beginning of the session, rocked with him and banged their heads together. When I spoke, he came back to sit on my lap, rubbed his penis, hooked his feet under the table and pushed and pulled it to and fro.

Comment. Although John's intention, it would seem, had been to triumph over the 'fish'-babies by defaecating them out of my inside, he appears to have lost the 'lady' in the process of expulsion. Alternatively, it might be that he felt himself pushed out of my inside. He appears to turn to faeces in order to fill up the emptiness inside him, but again gets worried that he had turned my inside into just a bottom. The sadistic rocking and head-banging collusion with Teddy came I think at a point where John felt the good lady to be gone beyond recall. When my voice brought him back to my lap, his masturbatory behaviour appeared as a last desperate effort to control me, stop me moving away. The nakedness of John's despair, the feeling of total loss of the mummy-lady seems here to have arisen from a lack of differentiation between the self and his object, between what he does inside his body and what he does to me externally. The material strongly suggests that this defaecation is concretely felt by him to be expelling babies out of my bottom as well as his own. Hence it might just as easily be himself as the others who have dropped out. My chair-seats were so absolutely identified with his bottom that they smell to him just like his trouser-seat. They do not offer any reassurance to the distressed child that I can survive externally as a top- and lap-mummy different from the destroyed internal bottom-mummy.

John's reality-testing is impaired because of his reliance on a single sense datum, his sense of smell in this instance. This ordering of his objects in terms of one sensual modality at a time was typical of John as of the other autistic children in our group. They appreciated highly the sensual qualities of an object, but were all nose, all ears, all eyes at different times. It occurs to me that this strict separation of the senses in the self might be the consequence of using the senses to separate and control parts of the mother one by one, to own her eyes, her ears exclusively; the conjunction of different sense organs may be felt as a togetherness of parts of the object which sets off murderous jealousy and so they are continually kept apart, and tend to function in isolation from each other. This suggests a connection between the autistic phenomena of sensual dissociation in the self and the less primitive obsessional separating of objects in order to control them. But such separation of sense data leaves John at the mercy of despair when a part of mother's body has been attacked, for he lacks the means for reality testing. In the session discussed above, the bottom literally fell out of John's existence, he lost my holding lap as well as his faeces and was not able to establish by touching or looking whether it still existed.

During the next few sessions he made some attempt to re establish his relationship to the sweets-breast, to sort out the smell-bottom with its faeces and smells from the taste-top with its analysis-milk. He engaged my hand in helping to put the sweets in a pile separate from that of the plasticine chunks. Yet it was probably significant of his confusion of zones that the sweets he brought were 'All Sorts', the kind which has black liquorice sandwiched between light colours.

His cough worsened over the next few days, so that he had to be kept in bed after the weekend. He wanted his mother rather than anyone else to nurse him which pleased her, and she felt in better contact with him than she had been since his infancy.

When John returned, he spoke with the old gruff voice, saying 'mooss' which sounded like a mixture of 'milz' and 'poohs' (his words for milk and faeces), and shook himself when he coughed as if to get rid of something bad inside him. His behaviour varied between snuggling up very close to me and banging his head violently with Teddy's. As soon as he saw a bird, his head dropped like a flower nipped from its stem. At the end of sessions, he went completely limp, forcing me to carry him down. His demeanour was pathetic, as if indicating that I was cutting him off from his life-line and abandoning him to be killed off by rivals and persecutors.

*The last two sessions before the holiday: getting in –
keeping out*

On the day before the holiday, John completely emptied out his drawer, bit the pencil points off, tipped out and rummaged amongst the spilled contents, bit the tangerine seeds he found in the wastepaper basket and tore the paper into shreds. He was very distressed when it was time to leave and tried to pull me back into the room. When the parents brought him the next day, they reported that John had cried inconsolably throughout most of the night, even when taken into their bed. He took my hand and pulled me upstairs, went straight to the drawer and took out the woman doll, two pencils and two balls. He rolled the balls gently towards the drawer and placed them inside. Then he rolled the pencils on top of the chest of drawers and when they dropped behind, he took my hand and indicated that I was to retrieve them; he examined their tops and bit off their points. He was 'talking' non-stop – lady, milz, flowers, aeroplanes – repeating the words he knew over and over again. He made the aeroplane fly and then examined its underside. Then he pulled my mouth open, looked inside and went to fetch the holiday-chart. He sat on my lap and listened carefully while I once more repeated 'lady here . . . lady gone . . . lady back again' explanations, pointing at each circle in turn. He let me go right through the chart and when I had finished, he produced the first whole sentence I had ever heard him speak: 'John must not go to the garden'. Then he sang softly, 'lady, lady, lady gone', in the way of a lullaby. This peaceful episode was suddenly shattered by his banging his head violently into mine, but he immediately cuddled up again. He repeated the banging and cuddling a number of times, allowed me to guide him down-stairs at the end of the session, and left in a very gentle mood.

Comment. After such ravaging attacks on the analyst's possessions, one would in other psychotic types of children expect a
fear of retaliation, great persecutory anxieties, an inability to face
the damaged object. Not so with John – his primal and overwhelming fear after such attacks was of loss and separation ; he
was not unable to face the damaged object (persecutory depression), but rather could not tolerate the possibility of irreparable
loss. When my reappearance assured him about my survival, he
made some attempt to restore the ball-breasts to me. But this
involved giving back the pencil-points/nipples too (combined
part-object), and at that his jealousy flared up and he could not
manage it. We see him struggling against banging his way in,
listening to daddy's voice telling him to keep out, not to intrude.
It is difficult to know to what extent he was able to internalize
an image of the therapist as a person, but at least the germ of the
idea is there. One can discern the wish to be able to take me,
undamaged like the balls, in and out of the drawer of his mind,
and thus to have my voice available to him when he needed the
comforting analytic music. It was surely this longing to be able
to do so, his failed attempts and struggles, which made this such
a moving session.

Thoughts about John's attempts to deal with the separation

We saw John trying to deal with the first holiday of his analysis
in a variety of ways:

(i) There was an initial unsuccessful attempt to conserve the
relationship to the sweets-breast in the face of jealousy of his rivals.

He attempted then to create some horizontal split, to divide
his object top and bottom between himself and his rivals. This
did not succeed either.

He tried to divert the aggression from the top to the bottom
and smash up the babies there; but at that point confusion set in.
He was no longer able to distinguish whether he had destroyed
the top or the bottom; whether he expelled the babies or was
himself expelled.

It was at this moment that John slumped into despair, and
experienced some sort of primitive catastrophic depressive anxiety of being lost, abandoned and forgotten.

Perhaps the failure to take in a containing object was at this stage no longer so much related to the absence of a concept of a mother with boundaries which can hold the baby and its fears, but rather to his intolerance of structure itself. Structure implied for John the presence of daddy-pencil guards who bar the entrance. What was the nature of these guards? Were they lion-daddies who stop the baby getting to mother's riches, even to her breasts when he needs them? Might this relate to mother's early illness when John had to be kept away from mother? Or was there a failure to relate to a feeding mother except by becoming the point-nipple, being the tongue-penis right inside? Such erotization of the relationship implies that being put down by me for the holiday would be felt by John as a betrayal, choosing daddy to replace him, being discarded and forgotten as a lover rather than being temporarily put down as a baby. This would fit John's behaviour at eighteen months when his parents went away. It was against a repetition of this experience of mutual expulsion that we seemed to struggle in the analysis.

The idea of being kept in mind may have gained some strength, for John seemed able to maintain the relationship and even make progress in this and subsequent holidays. The mother reported that he cried often in the first few days and was generally subdued. For the rest of the time he was in close contact with his mother and wished her to play with him and comfort him.

The first session after the Christmas holiday: insider or outsider – Daddy or John

John looked pale and rather dreamy but was jumping up and down on his mother's hand when I opened the door. He immediately took my outstretched hand and walked excitedly upstairs. He pressed paper and pencil into my hand, said 'aeroplane, aeroplane' and indicated the paper with some urgency. I understood that I was to draw and as soon as I had done so, he crossed the aeroplane picture out and smeared thick, black lines over it. He again asked me to draw an aeroplane and repeated his actions. He had always been preoccupied with aeroplanes but I had never before had to draw them, nor had there been any paper-work except in relation to the holiday chart. Therefore I interpreted that I was to produce this holiday aeroplane-daddy that had taken me away from John so that he could scratch it out and turn it into poohs. John then rolled the whole bunch of pencils on top of the chest of drawers, let them drop behind one by one and left them there. He rolled some plasticine sausages, left these on the table and pulled me by the lobe of the ear (twisting it in quite a torturous way) to the window, where he looked down onto the snow-covered ground. He pulled me to the couch, bounced up and down, laughing, and tried to pull me to lie next to him. When I refused to do so, he kicked his feet into my stomach, bounced and laughed again, pushed his feet up the wall, hung his head over the edge of the couch and said challengingly 'up'. I think some sound coming from outside may have disturbed him for he suddenly pulled me over to the window by the earlobe and gazed down. He looked around the room anxiously, hit his head with his hand, then banged the table furiously. I had the impression that 'daddy' banged him out of my inside and John in turn attacked me for containing this daddy and letting him take possession of me. When it was time, John said in a gruff voice: 'that's enough for you', and there was no doubt that 'daddy' was telling John he'd had his turn, it was time to get out. As we descended the steps John said 'down, down' and once outside he scooped up handfuls of snow and ate them.

During the next few sessions John's behaviour varied. In part, he seemed a circumspect invader trying to outwit the enemy, by smelling the stairs, looking around carefully, tapping the ground and walls on his arrival. In other ways he was establishing himself via the plasticine whip as a cruel overseer of the mummy, forcing entry and bouncing up and down on the couch in possessive triumph, only finally to relapse into despair at any sounds from outside. At the end of each session he became once more a furious outsider trying to bang his way in. The following will show how quickly John changed from one mood to the other and how liable he was to collapse into depression and despair.

Intrusion and collapse

John looked vacant when he arrived on the Monday of the second post-holiday week. He smelled the steps, put his head to the floor after tapping it, swooped on a bit of fluff in the corner, exclaiming 'aha, aha'. He examined the waste-paper basket, jabbed pencils into the key-holes of the other drawers, tried to push the whole chest over and then beat it with a long plasticine sausage. He bounced up and down excitedly; but stopped abruptly when he heard a child's voice in the street below. He made hissing noises and rolled his eyes inwards and then looked up towards the ceiling, perhaps as if he could change the child-in-the-street to a fly-on-the-ceiling. Then he danced around in circles, laughing more and more wildly and ended up stamping with all his might on the floral pattern of a green rug. Suddenly his face crumpled, his body sagged, and he staggered over to my chair, leaned against my leg and sucked his forearm; the triumphant war-dancer had from one moment to the next become a pathetic, lifeless infant. After a few minutes, John began twisting plasticine into tiny twigs and waved these about rather apathetically. He gazed out of the window, twisted first my ear-lobe, and then scratched his own. Moving slightly in the direction of the window to say 'go away' in a weak voice to the birds in the tree, he quickly came back to bury his head in my lap. I then became aware that he had defaecated. I think he must have done so when he stamped on the carpet. He asked to be lifted onto the window-sill, looked outside and then deeply into my eyes, wiped his hand over his bottom. He sniffed at some plasticine, bit it, threw it away, twisted another bit into tiny twigs, broke them in half, chewed some and spat them out again. When he saw his mother arriving in a chauffeur-driven car, he picked up a toy car and banged in into his head and then banged his head into the side of the couch.

Comment. I should like to discuss this session in some detail as the sequence of events clearly shows John's despair, his manic defences, and their failure. We see him arrive in a depressed mood, feeling suspicious, expecting 'daddy's' ominous presence in every corner of the room. He seems to be able to conquer this rival primarily with his faecal whip. This seems to set off an omnipotent episode in which my other babies are to be rolled out of sight and beyond ear-shot (both his and mine) by trampling and dancing on the carpet-part of mummy's body. But suddenly his omnipotence deserts him, his triumph over his rivals miscarries and it is he who is bereft.

The question arises: did he feel he had gone too far in his cruelty to my inside babies, overstepping the limits of my tolerance? The pleading with the birds to 'go away' would fit in with the idea that he is begging them not to provoke him by their presence into further murderous attacks. But when we remember the earlier episodes of the tip-up lorry, his frenzy after defaecating the 'babies' out before holiday, it might be thought that his manic excitement and expulsion of my contents resulted in 'mummy' falling out along with the babies. It looks as if John has little control over what he wants to retain or expel. He does not clearly distinguish between expelling his object, being the object expelling his rivals, and being himself expelled by his object. Consequently he despairingly turns to faecal food, as if this is all that is left to him – or, more likely, he feels compelled to eat his faeces in order to re-introject the maternal part-objects he has dropped out of his bottom. The sight of his mother and chauffeur aroused once again tremendous oedipal rivalry as if he were looking into this realm of combined objects from which he had been exiled. It drove him to despair and precipitated another attempt at banging his way in.

Through the looking-glass: 'roses, roses'

I had to cancel the Friday session of the following week because of minor illness. After this longer weekend John discovered the stained-glass windows above the stair landing. It was as if he were sucked up into the dark red roses which form part of the pattern. He went towards them with an expression of wonder and fascination, pressing his face against them. Even when I persuaded him to proceed further up the stairs, he continued to gaze back at them. He seemed pulled back as if by magnets, and I had to walk behind him to stop him falling.

Once in the room, he rummaged through the drawer and, apparently not finding what he wanted, pulled hard on the handles of the other drawers, making angry noises when they would not yield. He ran to me, pulled at the collar of my blouse and looked down inside, saying 'aha, aha'. He again cried angrily, made another attempt at pulling the drawers open and then found two buttons in his drawer and put one on top of the other.

He rolled some pencils briefly and after a glance at the 'daddy-chair', and the ceiling, swooped down on the waste-paper basket. He tipped its contents onto the couch, examined some tangerine peels and then placed these on the floor, alternating the convex and concave surfaces. He then wanted to be lifted up onto the window-sill, pushed me away while he pulled the curtain to and fro, hiding behind it. He threw some bits of plasticine towards the 'daddy-chair' in the corner, clenched his teeth as he swung the lamp to and fro; then he pushed and pulled me. Suddenly he said 'gone for walk' and fell back against my shoulder, crying. He put two fingers into his mouth, then threw himself, sobbing, into my arms and I found myself carrying him about like a baby.

When it was time to go, he ate some tangerine seeds, bit hard into an India-rubber, buried his teeth in the soap and flung it away into the basin. On his way down, he again peered deeply into the red roses.

Reflections on the changed nature of John's relationship

These examples of John's post-holiday play strongly suggest that he now felt himself much more to be outside and looking in to the combined mummy-daddy relationship. The holiday and the extended week-end have crushed a certain amount of omnipo-tence, of feeling able to tear open and take possession. No longer, as in the first term, does John's maternal object seem defence-less, her orifices open to intruders. The orifices seem to be less permeable and to have specific points of entry; his object now has a structure which resembles drawers with contents and nipple-knobs and holes to look through and see if you can pull out the daddy-penis-key nipple. Because of being more protected by the daddy door-keeper nipple, this mummy breast becomes for John more permanently owned by the 'daddy' and stimulates his curiosity as well as his wish to participate through voyeur-ism in the mummy's and daddy's union. The mesmerization by the red roses suggests high erotic excitement; he demands to get in, to possess himself of the light-breast, to get hold of the button-nipples, to throw the seed-babies out so that he can have an exciting swinging time with the lamp-breast mummy. He is both the baby, pulling and pushing the breast, and the nipple-tongue daddy who controls and excites it. But again his attempts miscarry; not for long is he able to maintain this idealized relationship with the rose lamp top. Was it daddy who came along and took mummy away 'for a walk'? Or did he feel that I would not stand his biting, pushing control and be 'gone'? Is he referring to his anxiety that whenever Mother 'goes for a walk' his greed has destroyed her? Whatever the phantasy, he then tried to split off his oral sadism onto the soap in order to preserve his idealized relationship with the rose-nipple.

At the taps

It was in the following session that John began playing with water, and this was to be his main preoccupation for the rest of the term. He used it first to wash his hair; then he examined and felt the pipe underneath the basin, tapped the floor as if to see where the drains were. He then splashed the water straight onto the floor and tried to rub it in. This kind of play developed into spilling larger and larger quantities onto the lino and trampling in the puddles. He also began spitting into my face, and this would always be followed by great excitement, jumping and dancing around in circles with eyes glinting with triumph. Occasionally, he glanced in a frightened way towards the corner 'daddy-chair'. On his way up, he looked gloatingly at the red roses of the window, stared at them and sometimes scratched them on his way down after the session. He also used the water for drinking but, after only one or two sips from the red beaker, he would throw the water high up into the air and drop the beaker on the floor. When the floor became too wet I stopped him and afterwards he kicked and threatened to return to eating plasticine. I felt that the setting of limits was important for him. I suspected that it meant to John that I would not allow myself to become an overflowing kind of toilet mummy. As the weeks went by, his play became wilder, his dancing more triumphant, and his play very repetitive. Although he behaved in a manic way with me, he often cried in the night at home.

Comment. What may have started as a relieving experience, using the water to clean his hair and his mind of bad thoughts, appears to have gone wrong, turned into something else. We saw him exploring the pipe-structure which might be thought of as the daddy-plumbing-penis that takes away mummy' s messes and tears, but he deliberately bypassed this daddy-pipe and put the wet onto the non-absorbent floor. The taps themselves were also appropriated in a way that changed their function. Was the jealousy aroused by the combined basin-and-pipe object impelling him to separate them? His excessive spitting and wetting and the growing feeling of despair which I experienced, convinced me that he was not utilizing the feeding and cleaning aspects of the taps but rather employing them as weapons, a perverse use of the nipples as penises to urinate into mummy. And at times he was quite frightened of a counter-attack, as when the water squirted up at him. His mother reported that he was now terrified of having his hair washed.

As time went on, the monotony of his play, his absorption in the drowning and spitting activities, his misuse of objects, evoked a growing despair in me and the feeling that we were locked in a non-growth-producing relationship. I thought that some confusion had arisen regarding the daddy and the nature of his relation to the mummy. Perhaps the teddy and the daddy had fused. He seemed concretely able to ejaculate his spit-tears into me, but this did not produce any relief. Rather the projection of his tears and depression seemed to encourage a sadistic and negativistic isolation that was unalloyed with any tenderness.

One week before the Easter holiday: 'all mine'

He brought Teddy to this Friday session, put him under his stomach and rocked with him. Then he turned the taps on, let them run, splashed about, squirted water for several minutes and, when I stopped him making too much of a mess, again rocked with Teddy. He turned the taps on again, but after a while they ran sparingly. He took my hand and when I did not succeed in making the water come out faster, he slapped the taps, clenched his teeth and banged his head into the side of the couch. He stood on the window-sill and made a mark with a brown pencil, high up on the wall by the window; he hid behind the curtain, scratched the wall and peeped out from time to time. Suddenly he cried and put his arms out to be lifted down.

He sat on my lap, held onto my earlobe and looked sadly into the distance.

I tried to go over the holiday-chart, which John had already been shown a number of times, but he pushed it away. He pulled frantically at the other children's drawers, saying 'mian, mian'. He filled two bowls, then a number of small cups, drank one after the other saying 'wait a minute'. Presently he tipped the bowl of water onto the floor, still holding on with his teeth and crawling on all fours. He ran to the corner chair, threw out the cushion and for the first time sat on it. He switched the lights on and off several times, saying 'mian, mian', then held the green pencil under the tap and bit off its point. At the end, he looked sad and slowly slid down the stairs on his bottom.

Comment. The impending holiday has brought the relation to the feeding mummy more to the fore; he seemed to feel that someone else was emptying the water-taps, perhaps an inside baby, and this set off his murderously jealous attacks on the mummy's body: head-banging, scratching and dirtying the wall-skin. He was furious that it was not all his, that he had to 'wait a minute' while other children had a turn, tipped out the contents in anger, bit and tore and tried in vain to unseat daddy from his position of being in control of mummy.

Two sessions before the Easter holiday

John came in, dragging a four-foot long branch. He looked pale, serious and intense. He beat the hall floor with his branch, then the stairs, and also the table, walls, door and little chair in the playroom. Then he tapped the windows and the Dimplex heater and laughed when it made a hollow sound. I interpreted how tormented he felt by jealousy of the babies who he thought were inside for the holiday, that he was trying to bang them out of me and that the hollow sound was like a baby crying out in pain. John dropped the branch, turned the taps on, rummaged through the drawer, impatient to find the red beaker. He threw away the soap and nail-brush at the basin, gulped down some water and threw the rest away, filled the beaker up again and drank some more, looking up at me. Turning on both taps, John then inserted the plug and, when the basin was nearly full, he scooped out handfuls of water to drink. I said that he was trying to empty out both taps as well as wanting to fill himself up before the holiday. He ran to the couch and bounced up and. down on it for several minutes looking gleefully at the corner chair. He suddenly flopped down, holding onto his ear and sucking his forearm, then looked up at me with a pathetic expression. He came over to me, sat on my lap and nuzzled into my breast. I said that his scooping out and jumping on the mummy left him with an empty mummy-breast inside, which had all the life bounced out of it, and that he came running back to me as the full-top-breast. He took all the pencils out of the drawer, threw them all down except the brown one which he used for tapping the windows. He stood on the window-sill, pulled the curtains but leaned his bottom against my shoulder. There was a man sweeping the path next door and John watched him and almost at once tapped the windows in rhythm with the backward and forward movement of the brush. I said that he could not stand seeing this daddy man and quickly made himself into the sweeper-daddy, sweeping all the leaf-babies out of the analysis-mummy.

When it was time to end the session, John cried angrily and then sadly. In the last pre-holiday session, he returned to massive pouring and continually sucked from his soaked shirt sleeves. Paper and colours had been dissolved in the water. There was a great deal of water on the floor, and he came to sit on my lap, looked down on the floor and said: 'hold tight' as if afraid of dropping and drowning in all the wet below, a kind of toilet-basin which might swallow him up.

John had been having frequent bouts of diarrhoea in the pre-holiday period, but this cleared before the break. During the holiday he began to use his potty for the first time, and was alternately excited and sad.

Thoughts about John's relationship during this term

In this second term, John no longer seemed intent on possessing and living inside the whole of mummy's body; there was a clearer differentiation between the top part and bottom part of mummy's body: the rose-lamp-tap-nipple-breast and the floor-toilet-bottom. He had settled most of the time for intruding and taking over the top. One could say that he was insatiable, but it was not clear whether he was taking more than he needed or just never got a satisfying drink inside him. He seemed to me to be hardly concerned with feeding from this tap-breast but rather with taking over the control of the supplies, wasting them, stopping others getting them, throwing the food away and using the flow for drowning and triumphing at times over mummy, at other times over the other babies. The tremendous jealousy of the union of breast and nipple made him separate them, getting daddy to join in the fun of urinating on mummy and at the same time, through plucking out the nipple, leaving mummy as an unplugged incontinent breast which resembled a leaky toilet. And so he was still left empty and in despair when it came to a separation, afraid of having drained the breast-mummy of her supplies, having bounced the life out of her stomach, afraid of her leaking away inside or sucking him down and drowning him in her toilet-lap.

Again he made a tremendous effort over the holiday to spare his mother from his intrusion and destructiveness. He began to leave his faeces and urine in the potty, instead of soiling himself. Why? Did he feel it was essential to retain the food-mummy and not let her leak away? Did he feel that in my absence it was essential to hold with all his might on to the good feeding mummy? Perhaps the preservation of the top breast-part of the mummy was now seen as contingent upon the proper employment of the bottom-toilet-part. That would be a major achievement indeed.

The first sessions after the Easter holiday: the raider

John did not look at me but, after the first few steps, pulled me eagerly upstairs. I noticed that he was making sucking movements. He had brought a long stick with him which he waved about and used for tapping the floor. He looked defiantly towards the daddy-chair and danced round in circles. He took his stick and, pushing it against the window-pane several times, said 'babies'; it was clear that he was squashing them like flies. Then he danced around, laughing excitedly. When he heard an aeroplane approaching, he leant against my knee, said 'naughty boy', pulled me off the chair, smelled it and looked anxiously up to the ceiling and down on the floor. He drank some water out of the red beaker and splashed the rest onto the floor. He took the pencils out of the drawer, tried alternatively to 'write' on the table with them and to bite the leads out. When the latter broke in his mouth, he cried in angry despair.

Next day John pulled a part off a trailing plant in the hall and dropped it in the room. He was chanting a broken line of a song, as he rummaged in the drawer. He chewed at some pencils, protesting angrily when he found their leads gone; he rummaged further with great vigour and angry exclamations, then stood and sucked his arm. He brought three little pieces of brown plasticine, indicated that I was to stick them together while he went searching through the waste-paper basket. He came to stand on my thighs, then gave a smile to the daddychair. He had continued chanting a melody which was clearly broken up into fragments. I said that he felt he had pulled and bitten the nipple-points out of the breasts and this made him feel that he had a broken mummy inside him, like the broken tune. He seemed to feel that it might have dropped out into the potty with his faeces and that I could put the pieces together again, just like the plasticine.

He hung his head low, smelled my legs, slapped them with increasing excitement. He got up, took a glue bottle and sucked its red teat-like top. Finding a little jug, he filled it from both taps and poured the water over his forehead. He put the floorcloth under the taps, whirled it on the floor and then stood sucking his arm, looking very sad ; then he took the soaked cloth and sucked that. He jumped onto the couch and bounced up and down wildly with his eyes almost closed. After a while, he took the dripping cloth, threw it up to the ceiling several times and blinked as it came down again. When it was time to go, he cried angrily and bit my hand.

Comment. The alliance with a tap-daddy who agrees to wet mummy had disappeared over the holiday. On the contrary, John seems to be defying daddy and to take renewed possession of mummy in a very oral way. With his magic stick, he feels able to rid her of the penises and babies, though he appears frightened of daddy's ominous presence, associated with smells. John's raiding of mummy's body, the biting off of the nipples, renders her breasts incontinent, so that he cannot distinguish them from his own buttocks or leaky bladder. Like himself they have no stopper to hold the fluid contents, are no better than a soaked floor-cloth nappy. John's behaviour suggests his despair about the destroyed, bitten-up breast, the loss of the good firm mummy; and it seemed to me that at the end he could hardly bear to look at this dripping cloth-ball and feared it would come crashing, pouring down on his head.

Abandoned to mindlessness

It was against the background of these happenings that I again 'lost' John. He would come with a vacant expression and dead-looking eyes, crawl slowly up the stairs, beat about with his stick, pour a beaker full of water onto the floor; then he would stand on the window-sill, spit down, run to the couch and spend the rest of the hour bouncing up and down on it. He jumped up, bounced back as on a trampoline, lifting his knees high, cossack fashion, bouncing endlessly, like a rubber ball in continuous motion, working himself up into a state of ecstasy. It seemed truly astounding to see this rather lifeless-looking child quite suddenly filled with energy, able to jump non-stop for ten minutes at a time. He would fall over but in a moment be back on his feet and continue bouncing, sometimes on his bottom instead of his feet, laughing loudly. He usually looked at me throughout. He would protest when it was time to go home, try to pull me back into the room but then jump quite gaily down the stairs.

How are we to understand this behaviour? It seemed near at hand to think of it as masturbatory play, intended to leave me feeling like the child excluded from the parents' exciting intercourse. It was tempting to think of it as a sadistic banging into my stomach to kick out the babies and other contents. Was it meant to subjugate me, to prevent the chauffeur-daddy from being inside me? Such interpretations seemed to miss the impression of a bird set free, in touch with a source of vitality, the springs of life-force itself. Nor did it feel as if sadism was the primary moving force, but rather an abandon to sensuousness; he seemed very related to my body, but perhaps united with it in a state beyond the bondage of time, unharnessed from the restraints of dividing barriers. This orgiastic sensuousness, which continued session after session, was quite impossible to break through with verbal interpolations. More than that, I felt that my senses were being painfully bombarded, my thoughts banged out of my head until I was tempted to follow him into a state of oblivion. I realized that I had to tear myself away mentally in order to be able to think at all. I felt John luring me into a state in which I would no longer be mind-full of his terrible feelings of emptiness and despair, but would mindlessly join him in a wild orgy of excitement, a dance of death paraded as an entree to unending life. The alternative seemed to be a terrible hopelessness of having to look at this dripping, perhaps bleeding floor-cloth object, to dissolve into tears at the sight of it.

If I was to regain John's mindful attention, it seemed that I would have to battle equally against the lure of his sensuousness and the threat of drowning in despair. I learnt from experience that I had to pit unflinching attention against his mindlessness, trying to hold him in with my voice, sing to him if necessary, in order to attract him back to the hope-mummy. It seemed that I had to represent an object who knew about the crushing pain which he was escaping, one who would stay with him in his grief, and not be dissolved by the corrosive quality of his despair.

'Naughty boy'

A fortnight later, John suddenly stopped his continuous bounc-ing. Mother had been telling him that a friend of hers and her child would be coming to stay with them. On his way up to the playroom John found a tiny ivy-leaf. He picked it up, twirled it, stared at it and waved it about. He took the red beaker, had two big gulps from it and threw the rest into the basin. He said 'lift up' and jumped down from the window-sill, holding onto my hands. He picked up the dust-pan and brush, bit and tore bunches of the bristles out with his teeth, then lay across the table, dangling his feet into my lap as he waved and twirled the bristles one by one. He turned to look at the corner-chair with a triumphant defiant expression, holding his hand in a characteris-tic upturned way which had become associated with cupping and owning the mummy-breast. He then spat on one hand.

After sitting for a while on my lap John spat on the floor to each side of the chair, then lay back in my arms, sucking his forearm. I said that he insisted on being my new baby, plucked and tore the hair-babies out of me and kept others away with his poison-spit. He made aeroplane-noises and then sat up, hung down to smell my legs, pulled my skirt up and smelled my knees. He spat some more, then returned to the tap for a long drink. After this, he lay on the window-sill, hit his head hard with the damaged brush, clenched his teeth, saying 'naughty boy; you are a naughty boy . . . open your mouth'. I took this to mean that he now felt that an angry, damaged mummy was knocking into his head and punishing him for tearing out and poisoning the other babies.

In the following session, John lay across the table pushing the hairs of the brush slowly to and fro, saying 'lady' in quite a sad way, and looked toward the big chair. He sat up, spat on one side then the other, hung his head in my lap and said 'naughty boy'. After slapping the little yellow chair opposite, spitting on it and rubbing the spit in, he looked up at the ceiling. Standing then on the window-sill, running to and fro, he jumped down stopping only to spit on the floor and suddenly came to push me off my chair in a state of great excitement. When I sat down again, John tried to push me off again. When I would not move, he knocked his head into my back and furiously into my stomach and knees, then his head into the table-top. He scooped out and splashed large quantities of water, knocked his head hard into the basin, took the brush, threw it up to the ceiling and shook with laughter when it came crashing down. Then he drank with his head deep in the cup and spat the water back inside, laughing uproariously. This was followed by more knocks into the side of the basin, and circling round the table. Then he lay across the table spitting on it and licking up the spit, knocking his head and banging it into my breast. He found some hairs on the floor, twisted and twirled them and went dancing around the table. When it was time, he bit my knee, and when I would not let him pull out a plant by the front door, he lay down on the pavement, fiercely banging his head on the stones.

Comment. The ferocity of John's jealousy had been exacerbated by the threat of a rival at home. He felt tormented, as if he would be totally abandoned. In turn he tormented me, pulling out the hairs and using them as hostage-babies, throwing away the brush-mummy-lady, spitting back the water-food. He was, so to speak, telling me that if I would not allow myself to be possessed and to be taken over by him, then that's the sort of John-child I would have to put up with. It is particularly interesting to note the various uses of head-banging. He did it with such tremendous force that it always surprised me to see that he was not covered in bruises. He used his head in these sessions to bang past the boundary and into my breast and stomach, in the same way that he earlier banged into the toy car and the side of the couch when he felt excluded. The smashing of his head at the end of sessions could be thought of as despair, but also as a means of tyrannizing over me, making himself into the hostage-baby that he would kill if I did not give in to his demands. But there was now also at times a new quality to the knocking of his head after he had made an attack on me: it was as if he was punishing himself for being 'naughty'.

Two days before the summer holiday: where is John?

John had been struggling in the intervening weeks with being either the outside, excluded baby or alternatively my new baby which needed to be carried about in mother's arms. This day he insisted on being carried upstairs and at once wanted to be lifted up to the window-sill. He tapped the panes with his knuckles, said 'in there' and 'wee-wee' as he watched the tree closest at hand swaying in the wind. He hopped up and down excitedly holding his penis, then drew the curtain around himself and started swaying in rhythm with the tree. From time to time he checked whether I was still there. Presently, he said in a far-off sounding voice: 'Where is John? Find him'. He came out from behind the curtain, spat on the window-sill and the floor and rubbed in the spit with the sole of his shoe. Then he jumped down with my help and took a drink from the red beaker, filled his mouth with water and spat it into the drawer. He subsequently pulled out every single item and flung it onto the floor.

Comment. John's attempts to be the new baby wrapped up in mummy's inside, or alternatively to be the daddy wee-wee dancing inside her, have failed. The realization that daddy will discover him and throw him out, leaves him once more enraged. If he cannot possess mummy's body, then he will not allow anything but wet and spit to fill her.

Two ways of dealing with depression: plugged-up – or collusion with Teddy

John arrived next morning looking pale and vacant. Mother told me that he had hardly slept; he had cried most of the night and nothing would comfort him. He put his arms up to me and as I carried him up he entwined my waist with his legs and feet. He wanted both taps turned on and watched them for a while. I said that he had been inconsolable because he felt he had emptied, spoiled and lost the good lady-breast. He got down, put the black stopper from the basin into his mouth and continued to watch the running water. The plug could be thought of as a stopper-nipple which was to stop him biting and spitting, to help him control the cruel-John babypart; and it might also have expressed the feeling of being plugged up with grief.

A few minutes later, however, John spat into my face, then went back on the window-sill. As he watched the branches of the tree waving in the wind, he jumped up and down excitedly. I spoke about a part of him that had felt utterly miserable at what it does to mummy' s body but that then a Teddy-part tells him to spit the tears into me. He thought thereby he could become the daddy and have fun again. He spat onto the floor, spat against the window-pane and then licked the spit back again as if it were delicious stuff, looking at me with a smirking expression. I said that Teddy is telling him that the thing to do with tears is to spit them into mummy because they taste so good when you lick them back from her. He came down, drank a little and threw beakers-full of water over the edge of the basin, laughing and dancing with excitement. He then turned the beaker upside-down, squirted water from both taps onto it and drank some of the water running off the top of the beaker. He was looking at me with an expression of defiance and glee. He splashed more water, danced and trampled in the puddle. When it was time to go home, John sucked the water off his wet shirt, and went off banging his head with Teddy.

During the first week of the holiday, John took liquids but refused to eat and was sleeping very badly. Both symptoms cleared up spontaneously, and he seemed quite happy for the rest of the holiday as long as he could have both mother and father to himself.

Summary of further treatment

We shall leave John at this point where we entered upon a prolonged period of hard struggle. The possessive jealousy in the good-John brought it into collusion with a cruel Teddy-part which added fierceness to his biting and scratching attacks and violence to his intrusiveness. At other times he was pathetic and remorseful, feeling that he should be stopped from hurting the mother and her babies. Often he was despairing about being left with an empty and lifeless object, and clung tenaciously to me. There were two features, however, which increasingly worried me and filled me with doubt about the prognosis. One was the negativism, which had begun to appear in the water-play and showed increasingly in the following term, as a deliberate misuse of objects in contempt and triumph. The other disturbing feature was his tenacious sensuality in relation to a piece of elastic which he endlessly twanged and waved in front of his eyes and my own. I felt it to be the musical aspect of my voice, my vocal chord as it were, which he had plucked out to render me mute with others and now made an object of fetishistic excitement (compare Chapter 7). This appropriation of a part of mummy's body seems to me to be intimately linked to John's possessiveness, his desire to have me to himself, and furthermore to prevent the conjunction of different parts of the internal mother's body, because any conjunction was felt as mummy-and-daddy parts coming together in a creative relationship excluding the baby-John. This evidence suggests that the fetishistic object is the result of the obsessional separating of objects into component parts and keeping a particular bit for exclusive enjoyment. As a result the building of objects suitable for dependence and identification is impeded. There is an impairment of reality testing of the 'common sense' type (W. R. Bion), formed from the conjoint evidence of the various senses. This seems to become a redundant function as a result of the attacks on linking (Bion) which have become widespread because of every link being seen as oedipal in significance at the most primitive part-object levels. Alternatively by dismantling his senses he could forestall recognition of the conjunctions.

It may well be questioned whether my technique was firm enough to help John experience me as a mummy who could resist his invasion. Although even in the first year I did not allow him to hurt me when it could be prevented, I was perhaps too compliant at times. Certainly, in the course of the second year, I felt that he was controlling me in a way that did not allow him to come to terms with my separate existence. I decided to tighten my technique; for instance I no longer lifted him up to the window-sill, knowing that he was quite capable of climbing up by himself. And although I did not resist his sitting on my lap, I no longer carried him, as the latter behaviour tended to be felt by him as my agreeing that he be my new baby. John made some progress in the following year and a half; he became fully toilet-trained, began to use toys more for the expression of his phantasies, and was able to tolerate other children sufficiently to make it possible for him to attend a special nursery. Yet progress was very slow and there were long phases of non-development. It was during one of these, that the parents gave up hope about analysis being the most useful way of furthering his development, and withdrew him from treatment.

Review: catastrophic depression

At the beginning of this chapter, I recalled my reluctance to 'pick up' John again in order to write about him because it meant reliving our painful experience together. Now, however, I find myself equally reluctant to bring the experience to an end. This no doubt is related to the richness of the material and the feeling of incompleteness when so many questions remain unanswered. But I am inclined to think that my unwillingness to 'put John down' has some specific significance in terms of this little boy's despair at being left. When I think of John, I still picture him primarily as a lost, sad little boy. Before leaving John, I would like to draw the threads of the clinical material together and delineate the sources of his depressive states and their relationship to mindlessness.

It was John's quality of forlornness which aroused compassion and made one feel that his tyrannical possessiveness was but a means of escaping from an appalling dread of being left alone. His persistent intrusiveness appeared to stem from the fear of the impending catastrophe of falling into an abyss if any space were to arise between him and the other person. Right from the first session he gave clear indications of his need to be held on to – indeed he had literally to be handed from one person to the next – otherwise he just collapsed. Behind his sturdy physical appearance there lurked a tiny infant, psychically unable to use his eyes, ears or nose to bridge the gap unless he was actually touching someone. Having not yet established either an external or internal relationship to an object which could be trusted to return, he dared not let it go. It made me feel that I should devote myself totally to this infant-John because he so clearly desired and needed my continuing presence. Yet his demands were so insatiable, insisting not only to be carried, but to become part and parcel of my physical and mental life, that I was driven to feel that one would have to bang the door shut to keep him out or alternatively that one longed for daddy's homecoming – or daddy-time – to be relieved of this baby. If I, seeing him but one brief hour five times a week, found him such a burden, what a terrible strain must the parents of such a child have to bear? It seemed humanly impossible to sustain enough energy, patience and tolerance of guilt and despair: guilt at ever putting him down, knowing that he would collapse into a helpless bundle or turn into a hyperactive, empty-minded shell. And the despair? That was due to the awareness that no amount of carrying him would alter anything, and the anxiety at finding no way to provide a satisfying experience for him which would sustain him over the briefest separation.

There were only rare occasions when anything approaching a normal feeding-situation could be said to exist between John and me, a live interchange of projection and introjection. Most of the time, John was unable to reach that stage of relating. Driven by his fear of loss, his endeavour was limited to hanging on and sticking himself to me. His characteristic positions were: on my lap, his back moulded against my chest or else perched on my arm, hanging on to my ear-lobe. This was John's contact with a live object while any spatial separation spelt abandonment. Mrs Esther Bick has described this as an adhesive identification, as the baby's very earliest way of relating to an object. My arms, my lap, my attention seemed to be the string which pulled John's mentality together. This corresponds to the function of the nipple in the baby's mouth which acts as a focus holding the baby together. At the moment of my withdrawal, John's mentality fell apart, or perhaps he let it passively do so rather than suffer utter hopelessness. Where another child might scream in rage or fear, John experienced his object as unreachable and so he gave up in despair.

Adhesive identity and its relationship to absence of mental development

His loss was all the more acute because it was impossible at such times to prepare him for separations. It was thus a sheer drop from a state of in-oneness to being torn off (Bick), or a part of him being torn away (Tustin), and abandoned to hopelessness. He always appeared pathetically helpless in the face of such a disaster, unable to prevent its occurrence other than by attempting to adhere to his object. If this was a primitive defence against loss, it was only of very temporary benefit, for it demands a changeless state, it takes no heed of the morrow, of the need to lay a foundation to lessen the agony of future separations. Its very essence is to cling and prevent the threat inherent in any change. Such fusion with an object implies becoming part of its substance rather than taking it in; at best identification is by mimicry. Introjection presupposes some object, however primitive, which is separate enough to be desired and taken in to the self rather than be affixed to. The difficulty with John at the beginning of treatment was the intolerance of even this amount of space between us. Similarly, he often could hardly be said to be playing with or using objects: he almost instantly became part of the twirling twig, the waving branch, the running water. I do not mean that he was in projective identification with such part-objects; it had a more primitive, gentle merging quality of sharing in their life rather than taking them over. At those times, I found myself unable to contact a part of John to talk to, a part of his mentality separate enough from his sensual experience to be able to pay attention and listen. Or put differently, a John who had sufficient distance from his object to be able to think about it. For thinking about means being outside, while, in a state of fusion, no perspective, no three-dimensional view, no thought can arise. As thought implies an absent breast (Bion), this had to be avoided at all costs. The price was that there was no mental life which could help him over the period of absence of the external object.

States of despair in the presence of the external object

John's demand for a state of in-oneness with his object brought about further states of despair. For a mother so open to invasion by John could just as readily be taken over by others. We need to distinguish this over-accessible mother with unprotected orifices from a more ordinary two-dimensional object. The latter would suggest a territory with properties of length and breadth and therefore capable of being shared out among competing parties. John's object was of a different nature. It had a skin you could tear into – as into the cushion – and the holes thus made seemed to be its only cavities. It provided no hiding place, no safety-net to hang onto should intruders appear. Any manifestations of life outside or inside this object automatically meant to John that he had fallen out of the hole and this space was now occupied by others. Such events drove him into a state of frenzy, compounded of murderous jealousy of his rivals and despair at being totally excluded.

This thin-skinned, porous object with which John was identified also made him extraordinarily sensitive to the events on the other side of mummy's skin, her internal world. It resulted in a most intimidating perceptiveness and monitoring of my states of mind. Moments of inattentiveness were immediately registered and led to fury as if my absent-mindedness showed my preoccupation with my internal babies or daddy. If I was weary he experienced me as rejecting, unwilling to bear his mental pain. States of depression or unwellness on my part left this sensitive child flooded with despair at having such a vulnerable maternal object, not strong enough to contain his destructiveness and pain. As treatment progressed and he established enough trust in my strength to risk attacking me directly, depressive pains, a fear of having emptied or destroyed me appeared more frequently. There remained however, a liability for depression to turn quickly into despair, experiencing the damaged object as irreparable. This was mainly related to John's possessiveness and jealousy which did not allow a daddy to be with mummy. And yet this irreparable object was too dreadful to contemplate and so John escaped once more into a state of mindlessness.

First steps in establishing a separate identity

One of the most dramatic steps forward was the sudden appre-ciation of the possibility of separateness without disaster. It was heralded by the reflection of sunlight on the wall. In one flash of insight, it appeared to establish in John's mind the concept of a mother whose internal space has been filled with some-thing related to the baby's needs instead of in competition with them. At one stroke, though alas temporarily, John the passive participant fused with his object, or alternatively the excluded outsider, became John the explorer. A space had arisen which he could traverse hopefully, his finger risking to make a path into my mouth and travel back into his own. This space between us, close enough to be creatively bridged, also gave birth to the idea of a claustrum inside me; and in identification, it allowed the idea of a claustrum inside himself. The achievement of a three-dimensional object, with internal space and thus capable of containment, meant that the foundation for mental develop-ment had been laid. Pain could now be projected into such a container, and in turn John could internalize an object which contained the frightened baby-John. This concept could be extended into that of a 'lady' separate from John and made it possible for him to have a space within his mind where he could store the memory of her voice and hold onto it in her absence. It even raised the possibility of contemplating the fourth dimen-sion, that of time units, of some sweets today and some tomor-row. It is puzzling why the patch of sunlight provided such an impetus to development when all other sights and sounds had merely served to make him feel excluded. I cannot help speculating that the bright spot brought back some memory in feeling from long ago, of a shining, glistening bottle-breast filled with the comforting milk he thirsted for. For once, inside and outside linked in a transparent way which brought home to him that mother and father could join together to enrich the baby rather than merely to exclude him.

From then onwards, we had evidence of John's increased capacity for introjection and retention, such as for instance his growing vocabulary. He struggled to close his own orifices and managed to achieve both bowel and bladder control. Some little headway was made towards this establishment of a structured object whose entrances were now more clearly differentiated and felt to be guarded by daddy. We need only remind ourselves of John's fascination with the rose windows to realize that he no longer just walked into or broke into his object but tried to spy through the key-holes into mummy and daddy's togetherness. But the tragedy of it was that being outside caused such torments of jealousy of daddy and inside babies that he was driven to tear down the boundary between us time and again and thus once more eliminated space.

Despair in the absence of the object and its relation to the arrest of mental development

John's continual fierce battle to gain exclusive control and possession of the maternal object, tearing, plucking, banging his way in, resulted in a defective object. He rendered his object incapable of being a container and holder of the vulnerable baby-John. He could not internalize an object which was not contaminated by being invaded and taken over by him. The nakedness to waves of despair of the lady-gone kind arise from his having no firm internal supportive situation to fall back on in the absence of the external object; and in turn, the absence of a strong enough internal object constantly reinforces his need to throw the whole of himself once more into his object – and so the cycle continues. Where identifications could take place (when mummy is temporarily allowed a daddy nipple-guard) they seem to be with impaired or restricted objects. For instance, the 'plug in the mouth' might have represented an identification with an object which was only allowed a wrong kind of combination, one that rendered it mute, though well closed to invaders.

Unable to get an internal mummy that can securely hold the frightened and pained aspects of him. If, John is left defenceless against worry and anxiety; his whole world easily collapses and he is exposed to the inrush of despair. Nor can he integrate the destructive aspects of his nature. And so he shifts hopelessly between something like the following states of mind: giving in to cruel parts, the John-Teddy combination of negativism and violence; when this has gone too far and is felt to make mummy cry, John's innate tenderness reasserts itself and we see him alternating between inconsolable grief and manic reparativeness. Another way of dealing with the depressive conflict appears to be the locking together of destructive and tender parts and he then is immobilized. He may either become anorexic to spare mummy's breasts, or mindlessly vacant to spare mummy's mind. Or finally, when overwhelmed by despair, John may return to Autism Proper, virtually throwing away his capacity for experiencing either pain or love.

Conclusion

It would seem that John has shown us that the very first step in mental development is the overcoming of the dread of losing the life-line of mother's nipple-breast-attention which holds the baby's mentality together. It appears to be an essential stage in the development of his separate identity, that the infant learns to tolerate a space between himself and mother in her presence. The baby who looks up into mother's eyes while at the breast and can smile at her after the nipple has left his mouth, has already achieved this degree of separateness. It is the first step in a long series of being able to be within one's own body/mind boundary which stretches from this momentary experience of separateness to being able to be alone and independent and eventually to that stage reached by only a few people, the capacity of the lone explorer far away physically or mentally, treading a path into unknown territory yet retaining an internal link to his loved object.

CHAPTER FIVE

Disturbed geography of the life-space in autism – Barry

Doreen Weddell

The process of establishing an internal world, with internal good objects, through introjective identification, as revealed in the psychoanalytic treatment of an adolescent boy, with a severe psychotic character structure, subsequent to an autistic state.

An object to be available for *helpful* projective identification of a part in distress, relieving that part and returning it to the self for integration (Bion) has to be an object with sufficient strength and resilience to withstand invasive projective identification (Bick) and the parasitic ensconcement of that part within the object (Meltzer). The material that illustrates this thesis, is taken from the analysis of an adolescent, who at the age of twelve was referred for treatment as he was ineducable, incapable of going to school and totally unsociable. When disturbed he was virtually unmanageable at home. As a young child he had been autistic, but this appeared to have been relieved at the age of six following treatment at the Hampstead Clinic. Subsequently a grossly psychotic character structure seemed to have become manifest. Barry's analysis was interrupted after nine years, when he was aged 21, at his own decision. It is material from the early stages of the analysis that will, I hope, illustrate how this child became able to establish an internal world that contained objects having functions and roles which allowed for the development of phantasy. This foundation allowed him ultimately to become healthier through introjective identification.

The phases of analysis to be described can be summarized as follows:

Phase 1 (nine months): aggression and monstrosity. The clinic, the treatment room, the analyst, were the focus of aggression, and Barry presented himself as an unbearable monster. The phase ended when Barry seemed to recognize the analyst as an object, that could be firm but was vulnerable, that had a skin which could be damaged, but could heal (Bick).

Phase 2 (ten months to two-and-a-half years): intrusive, violent projective identification. The floor, the walls, the furniture of the treatment room became the recipients of the patient's inner states of mind. This began to change when Barry could conceive of and draw a picture of an internal world that contained objects, equated with an internal family, who required space and privacy for appropriate functioning.

Phase 3 (two-and-a-half to three-and-a-half years): helpful projective identification. In this phase, Barry became able to recognize the analyst as an object that could relieve psychic pain and fear of dying. There was a change from aggression to affection, with in creasing co-operation and verbalization. The monstrosity began to recede, after Barry had cried to his mother: 'Now I know why I am ugly.'

Phase 4 (three to five years): dreams and introjective identification. The analytic process was clarified, through the patient's dreams, as he first began to go to school. The meaning of disturbed and healthy sleep emerged and there was evidence of the beginning of healthy introjective identification.

The material that now follows has been chosen because it seemed in accord with and to be confirmed by dreams occurring in the fourth phase of analysis. It is important to stress two points. One is that Barry's mode of communication was predominantly amorphous and mystifying. Initially it was mainly through   bodily activity, as in grimaces, the use of his hands and dramatic action in the session. Later he began to hum, to sing tunes without words, which I was expected to recognize. For years, verbalization was minimal, but punning and double entendre became frequent after the fifth year (1968), though with a continuing wish to mystify and control the analyst.

The second point is that throughout the early years of analysis, for the above reasons, I was largely dependent upon intuitive recognition of patterns of behaviour, and on countertransference for detection of the patient's moods and emotions. Constant supervision and latterly, retrospective discussions in the research seminar of the patient's drawings, verbalizations, dreams and transference behaviour have made it possible to write the chapter in this form.

Phase I (nine months)

A brief history of the patient is followed by an outline of the first two sessions, indicating the patient's conception of himself as a monster; something of the nature of the monstrosity and the accompanying early depressive anxiety. Events preceding and subsequent to the first holiday break are described, relating to the vulnerability of the patient's objects.

Brief history

Barry was an apparently normal baby at birth, though he cried a great deal until three months of age, when breastfeeding ceased. Solids were introduced with immediate success in the sense that he stopped screaming and put on weight. It was then noticed that he seemed to stare at objects and people with great intensity. He was slow to walk, being rather plump, and did not talk but was able to make his needs known quite clearly. However he was utterly intolerant of frustration of any kind and apparently ignored other children.

Barry's parents made great efforts to teach him to talk and by the age of six they seemed to have succeeded to a limited extent through treating him as if he were a deaf child. He learned a few words from a Swedish au pair girl, but was generally considered to be ineducable.

At that time he had a short period of psychoanalytical treatment at the Hampstead Clinic. In retrospect this would seem to have cured the actual autism, but a florid psychotic character development ensued.

Barry was referred for treatment again at the age of twelve. At this time he was incapable of going to school, and when disturbed, was almost unmanageable at home. He spent most of his waking hours in front of the television screen, eating his meals there, and seldom speaking to his parents. He was apparently responsive to firmness from his father and had a close, dependent relationship with his mother, in which he was lover-like though very dominating. She often found that she yielded to his blackmail and threats, to keep an uneasy peace for the sake of the father's work.

At the time of his referral, Barry's teeth required attention but he was quite unable to tolerate more than a few moments in the dentist's chair and no treatment had been possible.

First session

For simplification most of the interpretations, as they occurred, will be omitted. The main points that were understood or clarified later will be given at the end of the second session.

On first meeting Barry in the children's department of the London Clinic of Psychoanalysis there was a sense of shock; for a moment he appeared more like a gorilla than a boy; there was something monstrous, repulsive about the way he stood, head and chin jutted forward, arms hanging loosely, feet wide apart. He has a low forehead, penetrating eyes, and stood impassively, apparently looking at my abdomen while his mother turned up the cuffs of his jumper. After introductions, I told him where the treatment room was and immediately the picture changed. He set off down the corridor in a way that was reminiscent of the back view of a two-year-old waddling along in a bulky nappy: a two-year-old in the body of an obese twelve-year-old.

When I had told Barry that we were going to use Room 0, he said, 'Why 0? I suppose it's just a number'. In the treatment room, he stood looking at the table with the small toys on it, then sitting on the couch he said, 'They are babyish, I'm not a baby'; and after a pause, 'You have nerves, flesh and bones, that is all.' He was biting his lips and making half winks at me. While I was talking, he began to make movements with his hands that reminded me of the children's game with fingers: 'This is the church, this is the steeple, look inside at all the people.' Later when I had distinguished between inside and outside, he said that he was thinking of the dentist, that he needed a filling . . . he had had sore lips for two weeks. (This was perhaps a reference to having had a consultation with Dr Meltzer two weeks previously.) He referred to his previous analyst playing with him, then said 'You have a body!' waggling his thumb at me: 'You just fiddle'. He scratched the surface of the table: 'You have a mouth in front'. After a pause, 'A tail behind'. When I used the word 'penis', he said he 'didn't know that word'. He clicked his fingers together with a noise as if he were breaking them. He opened and shut his mouth while I was talking, showing his teeth in a somewhat wolf-like way, licking his lips and pulling little bits of skin off, eating them. He then began to make biting movements which appeared to be in reaction to my speaking. He continued to bite his lips, pull at his skin, his nose, his ears, making grimaces, and remained silent for the rest of the session, though I continued to interpret what I thought might be occurring.

Second session

Barry was somewhat reluctant to go down the corridor in front of me on the second day, but once in the treatment room, he sat on the couch. He looked me over from head to foot, then looked at the chest of drawers (where his and other children's things were kept). Slowly scanning the room again, he said, 'Where do you come from?' He looked round the room again, then at the doors saying, 'Who is there?' and 'Two in use!' (this seemed to indicate a fact that he had observed en route down the corridor, that there were two other treatment rooms in use). He began to stare in front of him, picking at his hands, his nails, scratching at a mark in his trousers at the knee. He made many grimaces, showed his teeth, first on one side and then the other. There was a smelly fart; he licked his lips, opened his mouth, gave little gasping noises, and held on to his wrist as if taking the pulse. He then held his hands tightly together, pulling them apart as if it were a violent and difficult action. His head and shoulders slowly became bowed and he gave an increasing impression of a little old man, as if despairing, staring at death. At this point great sympathy was evoked in me, as I interpreted; Barry sighed, but remained silent, head on one side – a kind of crucifixion figure. He began to grimace again, now holding himself as if he were in a straitjacket. He then began to play with his hands again, picking the dirt out of his finger nails, lapsing into the little old man posture, but this time even more hunched and deformed, so that it made me think of the Hunchback of Notre Dame.

When I said there were five minutes to the end of the session he asked, 'How many more ?', which I took as asking if I could stand seeing him again. When it was time he remained standing for a few moments by the couch, and looked back at me as he went through the door.

It was a very moving session in the countertransference, quite disturbing in its emotional intensity and the pathos of Barry's situation.

Comment. The contrast between these two sessions was most striking. In the first there was the totality of Barry's destructive ness, and in the second, the early depressive anxiety, despair, and what seemed to be the conception of himself as an unbearable monster. My impression was that he felt that only some kind of Christ figure could help him. I wish now to examine the behaviour in detail.

As I have said, the immediate impression that this was not a boy but a gorilla seemed to imply that there was confusion about his body image (later in the week Barry drew a picture of himself which he called a 'bamboon'). This was confirmed later in the analysis, when it became clear that he felt he could transform his body in various ways, making it huge, distorted, ugly. For many months he seemed to behave like an amorphous mass, a kind of shapeless lump, which he seemed to equate with faeces or the dirt that he so constantly scavenged and ate. It was only after three years of analysis that his posture gave evidence of bone structure and musculature. Barry slowly then became less repulsive and frightening. Later still, when he could lie on the couch, he seemed often strongly identified with an elephant as he got on and off the couch on his hands and knees. After some five years or so (1968) he was able to walk into the consulting room fairly erect and purposeful in manner.

Barry's eyes were important from the first glance at my abdomen, while in the waiting room; they were eyes that looked deep. In the countertransference I felt very invaded by their gaze. In the first session, they seemed to be the main organ of penetration and oral sadism, both getting inside and pillaging my body and mind. Later on it came to be seen how Barry's eyes functioned with terrible independence, as instruments of torture; as mirrors; in front, behind, above and below. The inside of the object seemed to become the space in which his eyes, as parts of himself, lived, explored and travelled around, demanding that they should see everything, go everywhere, without any restriction to this form of penetration. When later in the analysis the treatment room walls were covered with red chalk as if streaming with blood, the violence done to the object by such intruding eyes was clear. Still later his explorations of the London underground were carried out relentlessly; but more under the sway of a thirst for knowledge than brute possessiveness. Barry's TV watching also came to be seen as his way of monitoring and controlling my life, though prior to his analysis it appeared to have something of the function of sparing his parents, giving them some respite and time to themselves.

Barry's mouth seemed to function somewhat like his eyes, so that he referred to the body, the mouth, the tail, as if when be named them, they disappeared out of sight, down his throat. Later in the analysis, he would often appear to be eating what was being interpreted, as if words, ideas could be swallowed. Much later in the analysis something of this seemed to be confirmed when in one session he picked his nose, held his finger in front of my eyes with mucus hanging from it, saying, 'Minotaur has man'.

After a few days, he called the analyst Pig. Piggiewiggie became the baby and piggiewiggie wagga was masculine. Punning and double entendre were used a great deal in the latter part of the analysis.

Barry's fingers seemed to be used to convey how he felt he could turn an object inside-out, so that all the inside was immediately experienced as visible, and the problem of separation was indicated in the struggle to separate one hand from the other. The impression of his fingers being personified was very strong; they scratched, tore, ran all over the body; they picked the dirt out for him to eat and seemed, like his eyes, to get in everywhere. It was later recognized that his invasion by eyes and fingers produced the parasitized, eaten-up object by which he felt enveloped and possessed – the monster, the Hunchback, the little old man.

The fart that followed Barry's comment that two clinical rooms were in use, was the first indication of what later came to be seen as extreme possessiveness, often of murderous jealousy of other children, a 'sending them to the gas chamber'. This became the dominating theme during the next few weeks.

First term

Barry behaved in the clinic somewhat as his fingers and eyes had appeared to behave in the first two sessions. It became clear that the clinic was the analyst's body in a very concrete way. He rushed in and out of it, into and out of other rooms, down corridors, through fire doors, in a most possessive violent and disturbing way, as if he should be able to empty out, destroy or terrorize everyone he met. This, together with the violence of physical onslaught on his objects, on everything in the treatment room and, later still, the use of red chalk on the walls so that they appeared to be running with blood, gave rise to the conviction in my mind that he felt he could annihilate his objects. There also seemed to be a picture of my being equated with a helpless object, full of holes, without any structure or boundaries or ability to contain him (Bick).

This later picture was also linked in my mind with Barry's physical posture – giving the impression of a kind of amorphous mass that could also be equated with faeces, the dirt that he ate so voraciously. In the fifth year of analysis he verbalized: 'I cut you up in pieces and stick you back all over the place' (Bion's bizarre objects?).

The gorilla hands later became equated with octopus hands – masturbatory hands that were as constantly at his face in the session, pulling, picking, squeezing, tearing to pieces, as if by implication they were at his bottom between sessions.

In the fourth phase of analysis (4th year, 1966) the impressions of the first two sessions were confirmed in a dream in which *Barry saw in his box an effigy of himself, a death mask,* a horrible monster with four eyes, noses, ten legs and arms. At that point we were in touch with the full horror and despair of the little-old man-baby of the session just described.

Meanwhile during the first term of work there was very little verbalization, but the analyst questioned and interpreted, often quietly through the din, and this seemed to have a calming effect, with the analyst felt as a mother who knew how to wrap up and hold babies firmly.

It became clear that for Barry the problem of separating from his mother at the beginning of the session, and from the analyst at the end of the session, was such that it was necessary for his mother to bring him to the door of the treatment room, and to fetch him at the end of the session, instituting a kind of handing-over from one person to another. In this way some of the disturbance was contained in the treatment room. This had been achieved to some extent by the time the first holiday break occurred (Easter 1963).

Second term

On return from the first (Easter) holiday, Barry appeared at the outer door of the clinic, making a great commotion, bursting through and clawing at the inner glass doors in a manner reminiscent of the original gorilla-like impression. On this occasion the impression was horrific, but, as on the occasion of the first session, the young child showed through. Now it was a frantic, ravenous baby, clutching, grabbing, clawing in its eagerness to get to the breast. In the waiting room Barry swept all the papers to the floor, tore down the corridor, emptied everything out of his drawer on to the treatment room floor, and within minutes the walls were covered with red chalk. He made the chalks scratch and scream as he used them; they were dropped and then stamped on so that the floor was covered, red predominating; water was thrown over them and he rushed round the room putting red crosses on all the furniture, the couch and the pillows.

Barry succeeded in stamping on and flattening the waste paper basket, in between kicking toward the analyst's legs, grabbing at her hair, face and breasts. He then unwound a new roll of sellotape, trying to make it stick to various objects about the room, but eventually crunched it up in his hands and threw it down. By that time the worst of the onslaught seemed to have been expended. I had meanwhile been interpreting what I thought was happening. He threw the rag, wet and red, at me; held one of his lids as if he was going to gouge out the eye, then took off his jersey, hugging it to him. He then bent over the chest of drawers in the little-old-man way. After a few moments, he raised his tie to his lips as if kissing it, folded it over and laid his cheek on it in quite a moving way. Then he bit the tie violently several times, before leaving the session.

I did not know at that time that Barry had made my face bleed slightly when he had scratched it early in the session. The tender and depressive reaction after the holocaust was clearly a reminder of the second session, coupled with a spiteful revenge, arising from his possessiveness, as he bit the tie at the end of the session.

A week later, just before the next weekend break, there was again a great commotion as Barry came in. During the early part of the session there was a temper tantrum similar to that already described. This time he succeeded in slightly scratching my wrist. He looked at it momentarily and said, 'You talk too much'; peeped out of the corner of his eye, held his arms over his head, muttered away to himself – something about 'going on and on' – then turned to scratch some marks off the wall and left.

During the weekend Barry was apparently very wretched, not being able to sleep at night and had a slight temperature on the Monday. His mother phoned to enquire if she should bring him for treatment. When Barry saw me, he stared, then muttered something like, 'I thought you were . . .', turned to his mother, and said, 'Give Robin [his dog] some sugar'. He spent the early part of the session in the little-old-man pose of the second session, hut gradually seemed to revive as I talked. He moved his chair to the radiator, holding on first with one hand then with the other. He then took the chair to the table, moved into the corner, further away from where I was sitting. As I continued to interpret he began to look sleepy, put his head on his arms on the table and seemed to sleep briefly; he looked up quickly and then put his head back again, perhaps relieved that I was still there. I continued to talk; he looked up again and said : 'You disappear', then began to make preparations to leave.

On Tuesday as he went down the corridor in front of me, Barry twisted round and round, knocking into the walls and doors on either side, looking as if he felt sick and giddy, finally collapsing onto the chair as he got to the treatment room. After a time he wrote on the wall, 'I am herself ' and later, 'I am so glad to be here today'. He then drew on paper a house in red chalk, with what initially looked to me like flames or darts going in or out, but might have been indicating streams of blood. There were variations on this theme, on several sheets of paper.

Barry then began to stick these pieces of paper on the wall, with water, then with saliva. At first they were arranged in a square, then in a tall column. At the time it seemed to be a kind of plastering me up again – a kind of mending me with toilet paper (omnipotent reparation), after the destructive attacks which had actually made me bleed in the previous sessions.

Comment. Barry's mother subsequently told the managing psychiatrist that Barry had spent many hours during the holiday bandaging and unbandaging his legs, being much preoccupied with ambulances and hospitals. At the time when Barry actually succeeded in causing physical damage to me, I had thought it unfortunate, perhaps dangerous to progress and conducive to further sadism. Instead it seemed to have precipitated concern and depressive anxiety.

These sessions were subsequently recognized as concluding the first phase of analysis, with Barry's ability to accept the vulnerability of an object. The object, the analyst, now had a skin that could be damaged, but could heal, under the sticking plaster – the bandages – between sessions, in privacy (Bick).

Phase 2 (ten months to two-and-a-half years)

In this phase the floor, the walls, the furniture of the treatment room seemed to become equated with the surfaces of the object, as the representatives of the patient' s inner states. Barry continued to stick pieces of paper on the walls of the treatment room, whenever there had been an outburst of violence. On occasions, after the paper had been thoroughly soaked, squeezed and spread on to the wall, so that it would appear tissue thin, Barry would scratch it with a finger-nail, so that it would wrinkle, giving the appearance of skin caught by a jagged nail – a reminder of the earlier scratches. In the transference this gave rise to the impression on the one hand that Barry had the idea of something like a paper-thin object, vulnerable and sensitive; but on the other hand there was also evidence of his ability to accept the analyst as a firm object: firm in the face of threats of violence, and thus protective for Barry, other patients and herself. Some years later he verbalized, 'The most sensible thing you said was "no violence"'. Barry's bandaging and preoccupation with wounds now seemed to metamorphose into an overwhelming interest in orifices. He became preoccupied with entrances and exits as he began to draw, first on the floor, then on walls and eventually on paper. It was in the evolution of these drawings that the analytic firmness began to be structuralized.

Policemen appeared directing traffic in relation to one-way streets, protecting certain positions and marking where crimes had been committed. I was made aware that the crosses on the floor were policemen (blue chalk) and crimes (red chalk). Making the marks was accompanied by siren noises like those of ambulances, fire engines, police cars.

As this aspect of the transference developed, Barry's TV addiction was drawn into the sessions, first as 'Psychoanalytic T.V.', then as 'D.W.T.V'. The theme tunes were hummed by Barry, announcing the arrival of Z-car police and later Canadian Mounted Police. Subsequently 'God save the Queen' would be hummed when something like order seemed to be in the process of re-establishment during a session. Later in the analysis during the period when the confusion between breast and buttocks was in the forefront of the material, it appeared that the arbiter of the distinction between clean and dirty was Sigmund Freud, who had the role of the respected father. Once Barry had written Freud's name on the wall, the soiling and corrupting began to diminish in the session. In these ways it seemed to be clear, that when Barry felt I was a firm, well-supported, breast-mother-analyst, this meant that I was experienced as full of helpful, strong policeman-father-penises.

Meanwhile Barry became preoccupied with the inside of the body of the mother-analyst, her organs and her functions. There seemed to be some evidence in his drawings, that body organs were thought of as objects containing spaces, that could contain objects: babies appeared as well as policemen-penises. Eyes appeared to be inside the confused breast/genital-like objects as well as being outside looking in. This seemed connected with Barry's TV-watching and his way of actually monitoring the analyst's activities between sessions, for he lived quite close by the analyst's home.

Outside the analysis, Barry was spending a lot of time travelling around London on the underground now. I understood this to be related to identification with the father's penis in its exploring, detecting, protecting functions. Later on the route to and from the clinic seemed to be endowed by Barry (as shown in his drawings) with the significance of moving from one part of my body to another. He was in need of protection by policemen-penises himself, when he felt threatened by the intrusive robbers and murderers who happened to be in the news at the time, for instance the A6 murder.

At home at weekends Barry was still preoccupied, not so much with bandaging, but with plastering the walls of his room with posters, which he obtained from billposting men on the underground. This seemed to be a continuation of the omnipotent reparation at the end of the first phase, as already described.

As Barry's capacity for conceptualization improved he was able to indicate expressively in his drawing how he could recognize different states of mind and moods as they occurred, before analysis, during sessions, on leaving, with a return to chaos before the next session.

During the *second holiday* (the long summer break, 1963) Barry appeared to have had a short autistic phase, which began to recede as his parents brought him back to England. In returning to treatment, depressive anxiety was again marked after the initial onslaught similar to that after Easter; again the destructive episode seemed to act as a spur to increased co-operation. He began to draw on the walls rather than the floor, which somehow afforded a sense of relief and progress.

Some of these drawings together with the material accompanying them will now be given in sequence, covering a period of three weeks, from the middle of the winter term until the approaching Christmas holiday made itself felt. The line of interpretation is indicated not because it is necessarily seen as 'correct', but to complete the description of events in the playroom.

Thursday, 24 October 1963

Barry was seven minutes late, but then delayed further in the waiting room. After five minutes he came to the treatment room quietly with a pile of comics. He pushed the couch around and moved the table up close to the wall opposite the door. He was noisy and gave the impression that he was in a bad temper, which was interpreted in relation to being late, and his feeling that it was all the analyst's fault. He wrote on the wall, 'A-cars at 3 :45' (fifteen minutes after the beginning of the session).

He sat at the table and began to read the comics. There was some noise from the corridor and after a while some abdominal noises from the analyst. Barry made some grimaces, something like a pig snout and then what became known as his 'wolfmouth.' He wrote on the wall 'when I've finished reading', as if he was the breast-mother keeping some noisy children waiting. He seemed rather stuffed up as if he had a cold and sat picking at his nose, smearing the mucus on the table. He poked at the eye farthest from me; I interpreted his murderous jealousy of the greedy babies who were felt to have stolen the breast-mother-analyst while he had to wait, together with the idea that he could get rid of their noises by poking his eye out and that the mummy-analyst could be emptied of all the dead babies inside her by picking his nose. The analyst reminded him of a dream he had had earlier in the week in which the analyst was dead.

He then wrote on the wall 'everyone should die' and began to sing in a croaky voice. This was linked to the screaming-tillit-croaked baby-part that had thought the analyst was dead.

He got up and began to make 'jews'-harp' twanging noises and wrote on the wall 'A-cars 1, 2, 3' and beside them various registration numbers, from 1 to 10, then 'Dr Alive Dare' (a play on 'Dr Kildare') on the table. Turning the table up on its side he wrote 'welcome' and then on the wall opposite to the analyst he did a drawing which seemed to represent the route that he took from his home to the clinic. It also looked somewhat like a gun in a horizontal position with a sharp point at one end and a hand at the other, containing what might have been eyes. He made a variety of indistinguishable noises, and then wrote on the wall '10 cars all talking to each other on the radio', then 'we will do it again tomorrow'. This was thought to imply that he felt better protected by penis-policemen-fathers for the journey home with increased hope for the morrow.

Friday, 25 October 1963

Barry was again very noisy at the beginning of the session, gradually subsiding into humming, singing tunes that eventually became recognizable as a mixture of 'Rule Britannia', 'We plough the fields and scatter' and scraps of Christmas carols. Thus some hopefulness seemed to have remained from the previous session, that the rule of order might prevail, that one season would give way to another and that the possibility of fertility had not been destroyed between the two sessions.

(i)

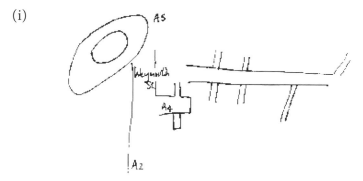

Barry then drew something on the wall (i) that was reminiscent of the previous day's diagram of the route to the clinic, though facing in the opposite direction. The A2, A4 and A5, seemed to indicate the presence of protective police-car penises that had guarded his safe arrival, just as they had prepared to see him safely home on Thursday. But the hint of crime and murder was also there, as an A6 motorway murder was in the news at that time.

(ii)

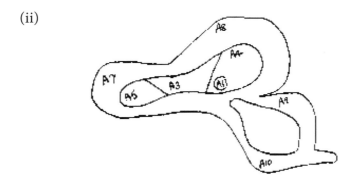

Barry then did another drawing (ii) which seemed to have much more to do with his feeling of being inside the body of the analyst during the session, with some confusion between breasts and uterus. Again there were A's, 1 to 10, but noticeably not A6.

(iii)

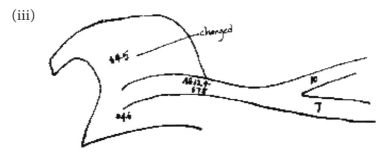

Towards the end of the session Barry drew something (iii) that appeared to be a combination of the Loch Ness Monster (already familiar in the analysis) and a duck (that could also be equated with an aspect of the previous drawing), and possibly the first indication of playing with words which was to be very prevalent later in the analysis, his and my 'little duck' (later he sometimes called me 'duckie'). The A45 and A46 were thought to be something to do with eyes and the numbers inside, AB 124678, and 9, 10, in the jaw part, again seemed to imply something to do with his feeling of being safely evacuated from the session. He said something about 'jumping into 45' (? fortified) and then 'it was different . . . it was A4A'. (? an eye for an eye). This was thought perhaps to be the danger, the kind of looking at the bottom that meant jumping into the lavatory and therefore the need for the

A-car daddies to protect him, fortify him, as well as to detect where the criminal parts of him had lodged.

As on the previous day he wrote 'Dr Alive Dare' and seemed to be breathing more easily than earlier in the session. He then threw the wet rag at me after having held up the one that was full of holes. He squeezed it out by the radiator and then over my chair. (I was standing at that moment). He went out, came back quickly, took the rag to wipe the door lintel, which he had smeared with dirty fingers, threw it back at me and left.

These two sessions were remarkable for the degree and quality of contact with the analyst throughout with much less mystification and far less violence than usual before the weekend.

Monday, 28 October 1963

Barry was on time and said, 'How is yourself. He looked around the room, puffing and blowing, pushed the couch towards me, pulled the mat and the rug towards himself, then ordered me to move and to put the mat under the rug on top of the table. He pushed the couch nearly to the door and put the chair on top of it. He then turned the table sideways on and wrote on it 'A-cars' and later 'thief'. On the floor he drew something which seemed to become a pedestrian crossing, and he drew a kind of barricade round the chair on which the analyst was sitting, saying, 'Don't move'.

Barry then began to draw on the walls (iv).

(iv)

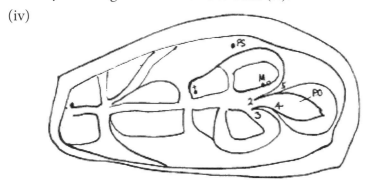

After a fair amount of rubbing out, something like a map again seemed to emerge. This time it was eventually enclosed in an ellipse, so that it began to look more like a swaddled baby. There were various markings on it. PS was thought to be an eye, monitoring what seemed to be the genitals. PO was possibly a contraceptive (post office = French letter). M, 2345 were thought perhaps to be linked with his thief-fingers, and an acknowledgment of his masturbation. The cross could have been the bitten nipple, the Christ-nipple, required to sacrifice itself to save him, as referred to in the second session, linked with the 'bandaging-up' after making the analyst bleed.

In the drawings, eyes, breasts, genitals and skeleton of the approaching Christmas holiday-baby, all seemed to be in process of being differentiated out, with some perception of internal space, of an object within an object. All were under the influence of eyes felt to be able to penetrate into the body and perhaps with something of the greed and devouring quality experienced by the analyst in the first and in many subsequent sessions.

(I had heard that the Z-car series on television – on which the A-cars, analysis-cars, were based – had been concerned that particular week with a thief breaking into a church, and then double-dealing with his companions. This was thought to be the link with the 'thief' earlier in the session.)

Barry then hummed the harvest tune of 'We plough the fields and scatter', scribbling in green and red on the wall. There were only little pieces of chalk, and he held them up reproachfully. He pressed very hard on them so that pieces broke off and littered the floor. This was interpreted in relation to the weekend and the analyst-daddy who was accused of stealing the good mummy-breast, leaving the baby with only the crumb-faeces to eat. He began to march up and down in Nazi fashion with much farting, which was interpreted as his wishing to claim that I was the bad, murderous Hitler-daddy. Clearly it was a baby-part of himself that wished to murder, to gas my Jew-baby children, out of greed and jealousy.

He began to use red chalk and to rub out, in such a way that the walls again looked bloody. He wrote 'no escape', making the chalk shriek on the wall. Barry then wrote on the table, 'Tomorrow Miss Weddell. She's been caught. Sent to prison', squatting as he did so. This was interpreted again in relation to the weekend masturbation, the resulting horrors and the dream in which he had seen the analyst dead. Later it came to be seen that 'in prison' meant being incarcerated in his rectum (his squatting).

In the last minutes of the session there were three drawings (v) which again seemed to indicate something of the way he experienced the session and the process of leaving. The first one (a) appeared to be something of a combination of a policeman figure, the Swastika, the Union jack, the Crucifixion and his route home. In the second one (b) something in the form of propulsion and expulsion seemed indicated as well. The last one (c) could have had something to do with musical scores and his humming, but on this occasion it was taken to refer to telegraph wires, not so much the radio cars talking to each other (as in the Friday session) but the protective aspect of the telephone with its reference to the possibility to contact the analyst if necessary.

(v)

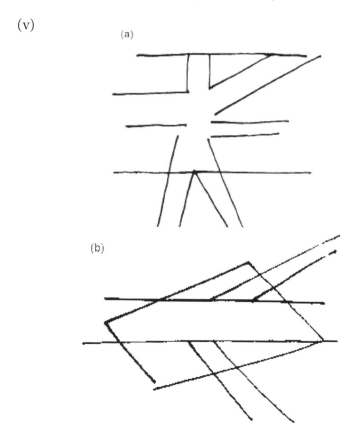

(a)

(b)

(c)

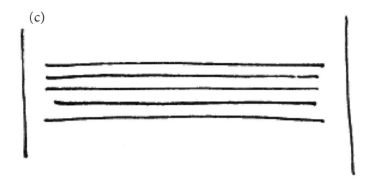

Tuesday, 29 October 1963

Barry was a few minutes late. He put the light on in the corner and, in the treatment room, made a great row with the table and chairs, moving them about in a way that forced me to move about as well. He turned the tap on, but there was not much water coming out. When there was quite a lot of noise coming from other children outside Barry reacted with banging, burring noises as if he was using a vacuum cleaner to get rid of the noisy babies. He pushed the couch around with much noise and, moving the table, said, 'It should be like this, in the corner.' This suggested that there should be a great distance between us two. He then wrote on the wall in red chalk 'A-cars at 3:40' and sat reading comics. He kept touching his nose which again seemed congested. He made his 'wolf ' mouth, 'pig' mouth and 'bone-crunching' noise with his fingers. When I interpreted that he felt that he had eaten me up and was crunching my bones, he coughed and choked, then put his finger to his eye. I suggested that he felt that what I said stuck in his throat and then got into his eye. He went on coughing which I took up as sicking up the bad stuff, the faeces babies that the scavenging vacuum mouth had been devouring, making links with the previous session (robbing the church?), the masturbation of the weekend and the previous night perhaps. He coughed again, brought up some phlegm, which he swallowed and then seemed to breathe more easily.

Barry then got up and drew (vi) on the wall with red chalk, something which again as it evolved seemed at first to be eyes, then breasts, possibly a uterus, later a penis and scrotum with something like a baby in each compartment. He changed the chalk to blue and connected the two areas, calling it a 'bridge', making the whole drawing look more like a pair of spectacles. It suggested the phantasy of his being able to see the other babies inside the analytic breast.

(vi)

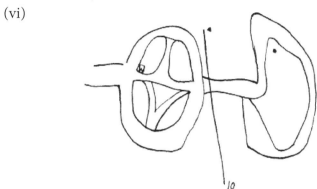

There seemed to be some beginnings of a distinction between top and bottom babies in the first area; a kind of simultaneous top and bottom looking. (Later in the analysis he would look up at me with one eye and down at my abdomen with the other – quite an experience in the countertransference.

In this session Barry then said something about, 'Thief goes to shop at noon. Weddell's shop at 3.30'. This was taken as his acknowledgment of masturbation, which involved a stealing relationship to the analyst. Meanwhile there was more about 'A-cars' and then he wrote 'part I' on the wall and underneath, 'part II'. As he left, he said: 'Stop talking, or I will eat you, fish-face'. He told the office secretary as he went out 'not to leave her gloves about' as if he was equating himself with the detective father warning about a thief.

Wednesday, 30 October 1963

Barry was on time and began by arranging the room, directing that I should sit by the door, which was interpreted as the need to have me as the policeman-daddy that would stop the intruders. When he began to write on the walls, I questioned why he had

to use the walls when paper was provided on the table. He said
when he wanted to use the paper he would do so (characteristic
of his extreme need to be in control of all activities).

(vii)

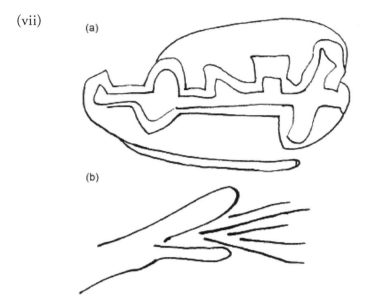

(a)

(b)

He did a big drawing (vii) on the wall opposite me. At first it
seemed like a face, then something like highways again appeared;
then it became something like a diagram of a chest, possibly
linked with his coughing. Eventually the drawing finished (a)
with something that seemed rather like a picture of a body, a
backbone, and perhaps the spinal cord and a long penis which
seemed to be equated with the breast-like structure. Perhaps it
was indicating the connection between penis and nipple as if
they were all one long tube. In the middle of doing this there
was something like the date 'Nov. the 3lst' and something like
'the 11th month' and 'the 29th'. I thought it was something to
do with the approach of Christmas and the holiday dates and
when he would return. There was then another drawing of something that looked like the head of a snake with five fangs coming
out (b). I talked again about the first picture and the drawing of
nipple and penis as if they could feed each other and linked this
with the five fingers in the baby mouth and the fingers that went
from mouth to bottom. The drawing seemed to indicate that his

baby-part was confused or identified with the breast and with the baby-in-the-breast.

There was then more about 'A-cars' and about 'boundaries' which were drawn out on the floor. At one point ten minutes before the end of the session it seemed as if he was about to leave but then he drew some roads in red and said something about the alphabet, 'new cars' and 'postponed' leaving at the correct time. It had been a session filled with his domineering and mystification.

Thursday, 31 October 1963

He was on time and by himself and said that the room should be ready for him, as he would like it. He wanted me to sit in front of the chest of drawers and he piled everything else on to the couch. The rug was rolled up and then he started to draw on the wall opposite me (viii).

(vi

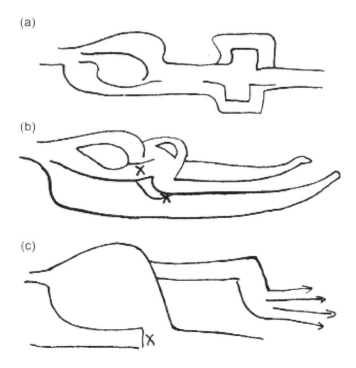

(a)

(b)

(c)

Again it looked (a) rather like a head of a snake, this time facing towards the left, with something perhaps like an eye or uterus or breast and again something of the pattern of the route to the clinic. 'PTV Times' was written on the wall and then he started to write on the paper and used four sheets, held them up to me, and wrote on the wall 'PTV Times, out on Fri. twopence. Programme Nov. 4th to 8th' and then this was drawn up on the wall first of all vertically, then horizontally; some more drawing on the paper and then back to the wall. He made a drawing (b) in which he said 'the roads' but these looked something like two fishes, one with an eye, two heads being somewhat like breasts, one with a nipple and the tail ends being penis-like. There were two marks in them, two crosses which seemed to be an indication that the passages in the roads were not to be gone into, so that there seemed to be recognition of the danger of intruding into the breast or into the uterus-ovary, fallopian tubes, with some kind of differentiation between penis and vagina. (c) There was quite a deal of farting during this part of the drawing. He stayed to the end and again daubed up the doors with red chalk which made me think of Herod's slaughter of the Innocents, the surviving babies, and the starving babies in relation to the Christmas holidays.

Friday, 1 November 1963

Barry was on time, making 'Huckleberry Hound' noises and read comics for a while. He poked at his eye, then wrote 'piggy, wiggy, wogger' on the wall, made grimaces and then did a little dance, as if to make me laugh. He looked at me and pulled something out of his eyes and then seemed to be trying to pull something out of his ears. He drew on the wall something that seemed to be an eye, but rather an empty one. On the other wall 'A-cars on Monday' and then something about 'February' which I interpreted as his wish to avoid Christmas. Then 'Harry Worth' and 'roads and road users'. He several times began a drawing, rubbed it out and then wrote 'postponed', then 'RCMP' then 'Hillman cars' and 'February', then back to 'RCMP' and began to march up and down singing the tune of 'Rule Britannia' and 'The Royal Canadian Mounted Police'. At other times there seemed to be something of the tune of 'Hector and Alexander'. He wrote 'Nov. the 4th to March the 11th. 4 month run', which I again took up as leaving Christmas out, making the holidays nonexistent. He made a hole in the rag, rolled up the mat and the rug, putting them on the couch. The writing on the wall was very big and as high as he could reach. He took a swipe at me with the rag and wrote 'can die' then 'PTV Times' joined with something like an eagle and a robin and then said, 'No change till Feb. Stranger might come in'. He sang at the door but went up the corridor quietly.

Monday, 4 November 1963

In this Monday session he was again violent. There was a lot of disturbance but the drawings (ix) seemed at first to be four men, who eventually became something like epaulets with crosses and v's on them. Eventually they were called 'prairie privates'.

(ix)

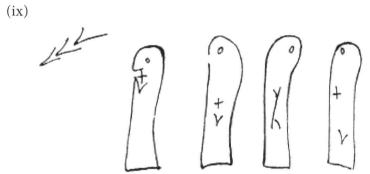

There was something about a 'Mr. McHail' and a 'Mr. McHailson' and he drew all over the floor and spilt the chalks and stamped on them and made a great deal of mess. He succeeded in kicking my legs, slightly scratching my face and then kicked the doors of the other treatment rooms as he left. The secretary told me later that he went in to see her, wishing to know all about the other children and said, 'How many does the pig have?' She told him to ask me. So he seemed to be beginning to be able to distinguish between internal babies and external patients.

On Tuesday, the next day, he was still rather disturbed but did a drawing (x). It was again something like a uterus/breast. He put

(x)

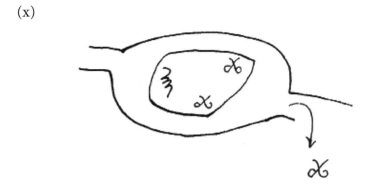

a big red mark in it, saying 'fire burning here', and several crossed swords – the map symbol for battles. Eventually there seemed to be an exit at one end. (At the clinic there is a fire door at one end near to the room we used.)

Thursday, 7 November 1963

He was early and said he 'had a lot to do'. He drew (xi) something that looked like a lot of continuous concentric circles but perhaps like an ammonite fossil; but then it seemed to be related to the mine disaster in the news that day. It made me think of

(xi)

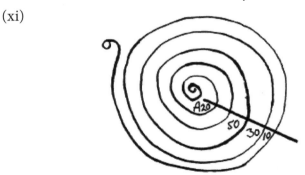

something like a geological survey with depths and how far down the miners were. It became a bit more like the bull's eye and his behaviour now suggested the question of the miners being rescued. He swayed several times in the session as if he were being gassed or suffocated, nearly falling over, lurching from one wall to the other at one point, as if he were a trapped miner.

In the session of Friday 8 November, there was a drawing something like the old woman in the shoe, the shoe part looking also like Noah' s Ark with a big eye and darts coming out of it, as if to represent watching various places in this shoe marked 'XI, X2, X3'.

(xii)

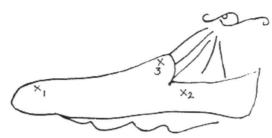

He asked me 'how do you spell penis?' in this session and then talked about 'Miss World 1963' and said, 'Miss Weddell has two golden tortollistics' and made a cross on the table with the rag and then wrote 'R C M P' down the middle of the table.

The possibility of internal babies being protected and rescued, and allowed to live even if a nuisance, seemed much more in evidence.

In the Monday session, 11 November, there was a drawing (xiii) of a brain which seemed to have in it something like a poking-in hand of four fingers. (He had often grabbed at my hair and poked at my face).

(xiii)

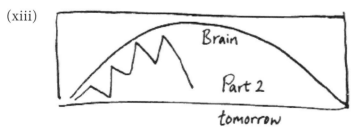

Tuesday, 12 November 1963

This was a very important session and central to this section.Barry seemed to be very disturbed at the beginning again and talked about 'Dr K's child' and there seemed to be trouble about the children in the other rooms. He was scratching and clawing at me and dragging things around, kicking at me and I had to stand up and move around the room to protect myself. He went out and took a lavatory cloth from one lavatory, came back and threw it at me, took it out again and brought another one in, went out and rubbed out the lines and mess which he bad earlier daubed on the door-letters of the other rooms. At the top of the corridor he made a lot of noise outside the waiting room and the office.

His mother eventually brought him down to the treatment room again. There was still a great deal of noise and I mainly interpreted the hatred of the father's work and influence, of the internal daddy who protected the babies from the murderers. He wrote on the table and on the wall and moved the couch to a different position and eventually wrote on the wall 'Miss W, TV, P T V' and 'Cast'. This was written in a horizontal manner. Next 'Miss W, herself, sister, office girl, brother Dr. Kalfman, father Dr. Meltzer, servant Sigmund Freud'; then he took out the 'servant' and 'Sigmund Freud' was a 'visitor'; then he wrote 'Drs. only, Men at work' and then he drew (xiv) something that looked a bit like a tooth but wrote in it 'Castle' with a moat underneath it, and a halo-like ellipse on top. This may have been a reference to his learning from his mother that I still worked at the Cassel Hospital.
(xiv)

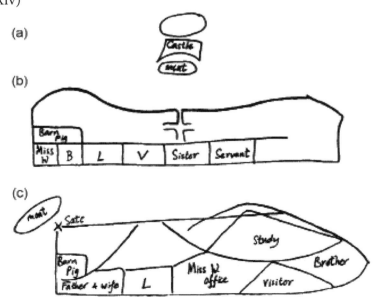

(a)

(b)

(c)

Then he drew something (b) that looked a bit like a coffin with a sort of headpiece at one end and a sloping piece at the other with a central cross on it and along the bottom there were divisions, perhaps like rooms in an L-shape, the double bit being on the left hand side underneath the head-piece. At the top was 'Barn pig' and underneath these smaller rooms 'Miss W., B, L, V, Sister, servant'. It was not clear what 'B L V' stood for at that point but I thought it was probably children. Then another drawing (c) was done still looking somewhat coffin-shaped. Again there was something called 'moat' at the left and he said, 'very deep'. The gate was nearest to the moat and then in a sort of triangular bit at one end was 'Barn pig' and 'food' and underneath this 'father and wife' and again 'L' which this time seemed more clearly to be the lavatory. Other spaces were labelled 'Miss W', 'Office', 'visitor', and 'brother', and 'study'.

These drawings were thought to represent the beginnings of Barry's ability to recognize the existence of an internal world, that contained objects which were equated with a family and thus a situation in which phantasy could develop. The drawings had aspects that could be linked with experience both of his own family and with that of the analysis, as there was something about it that conformed to the layout of the clinic and of the furniture in the treatment room. I felt that progress in allowing the mother internal space for her babies, guarded by R.C.M.P. daddy-penises, enabled Barry to experience himself with an internal space as well. Perhaps I, too, was allowed a room in his life-space and a place to study, implying that he recognized my need for time, place and privacy for study, to think about his material.

Summary. It was only in retrospect with the help of the dreams of the fourth phase of the analysis, that the significance attributed to these drawings accrued conviction. The manner of presentation is intended to help the reader to share this experience of prolonged uncertainty.

This material has been given in considerable detail, together with the drawings, because it seems to give an accurate picture of the work occurring at this phase of the analysis. It is meant to show how this child during ten months of analysis began to develop the capacity for conceptualizing distinctions between himself and his object; to recognize something of the nature of the object in physical terms and in terms of psychic geography as well. This allowed for internal and external spaces and distances between objects and within objects.

As the confusions were sorted out so the conceptualization of roles and relationships between objects, internally and externally, developed and with that the recognition of work and play, public and private (drawing xiv).

Once this was achieved it could be said that Barry now had an internal world in which it was possible by means of the transference to detect the changing geographical arrangements and the related phantasies and anxieties. With some conviction one could discern whether he was inside a part- or whole object; inside looking out or outside looking in; at the breast; on the pot; on the lap looking up or looking down; on the floor peeping up at mummy's bottom, etc.

It may be worth stressing again that the ideas and impressions, as described in the last few pages, were usually very tentative during the session and only became clearer in retrospect and subsequently clarified with the patient as occasion arose. Such a procedure probably contributed to Barry's recognition of the need for study.

The projective identifications of this phase of the analysis were, however, still mainly violent and intrusive in the sense of piercing, robbing the mother-analyst's body and mind in a manner experienced as violent and exhausting in the countertransference. This began to change and, in the third phase, helpful projective identification began to emerge.

Phase 3 (two-and-a-half to three-and-a-half years)

Synopsis. In the third year of analysis, death was experienced as 'the light going out of the show'. Zonal confusions continued to be sorted out, persecutory anxiety was sufficiently reduced to allow for dental treatment to occur. At the end of the period, drawings again appear and are seen as indicating the patient' s ability to appreciate his changing states of mind, before, between, and during sessions.

In this period, *aggression began to give way to affection* and the analyst seemed to be recognized as an object, as a breast, which could receive projective identifications and relieve Barry's baby-part of pain and fear of dying.

Three external events impinged on Barry's analysis during the first quarter of the third year. The first was the death of a TV star who had been a clever artist, talking rapidly as he drew graphic impressions of people and events. He was also quite a talented singer. Only in retrospect was it possible to link the change in Barry's material with this event. For the best part of three months Barry neither drew nor sang. Meanwhile a second factor, the terminal illness of Sir Winston Churchill, began to impinge. Initially Barry seemed to be mainly concerned with Lady Churchill and her bedside vigil. For days he sat on top of the table with his back to me, reading for most of the session. On one occasion he read aloud briefly, clearly and well from a treasured book, then dropped his head on his arms as if going to sleep. On the day that Churchill's death was announced, Barry spent much of the session with his head on his arms, and seemed to be projecting sleepiness strongly, as if the whole world were to go to sleep and as if sleep were equated with death. The weather at this time was very cold and there was snow. On the day of the funeral Barry was again preoccupied with the vigil, occasionally marching around as if changing the guard over the coffin. (Some four years later, when there were some falls of snow, Barry found it quite impossible to get to analysis; again the world was felt to be dead, and even speaking to the analyst on the phone did not help – 'it might have been a recording' – so concrete was the experience equated with the death of the breast.)

The third bit of reality to impinge was an appointment that had been made for Barry to see a dentist with the possibility of an anaesthetic having to be administered. Barry continued to be silent during this period, reading or writing out programmes, using a great deal of paper. On one or two occasions he appeared to be suddenly overpowered by sleep. As the time drew nearer for his dental treatment he became more occupied with numbers and an infinite variety of permutations, for example:

2 2 4 8 x 2 = 32
0132
4403
7799
32 22 29 40
36 60 40 100

This was thought to be connected with the equating of teeth with children and with ageing. When this was interpreted a week before the event (not for the first time) Barry said in a sing-song voice 'Bee bee see' (baby see) '3, 4, 5', while writing BBC 3. The next session dramatically ended the silent period.

Wednesday, 3 February 1965

There was a lot of commotion in the corridor and Barry did not wait for me to go to the waiting room but came towards me and other children in the corridor in a rather threatening manner. In the treatment room he began talking at once, very urgently, a great flow of words: 'There is a pig breast. The house is the pig breast. There are penises and children everywhere.' He was walking round and round the room saying 'This is a penis. This is a child. This is a penis. This is a child. A baby. The whole room is a breast'. The names of things changed as he went round, so that what had been a breast at one point became a baby the next time he passed round. I interpreted that I thought it was very confusing for the big boy part when the baby part saw things in this way, that everything seemed interchangeable.

He agreed and said 'The floor that you walk on, that's a penis or is it a baby?' in a questioning manner. He then drew on the wall (xv), saying, 'The penis is like the breast. The breast is the penis. The penis looks like this magnified'. In the first drawing, 'These are the babies, 24 nipples equals one baby, 48 babies equals one penis, 40 penises equals one breast'. He seemed to alter the places of the nipples, which also looked a bit like teeth, in several drawings, like the one in which the penis is a kind of tooth going into the circle as the breast. He then interrupted and said, 'Now it is time for a commercial but back in a moment'. There was then a further interruption and then rather sadly, 'No breast, only penises'.

(xv)

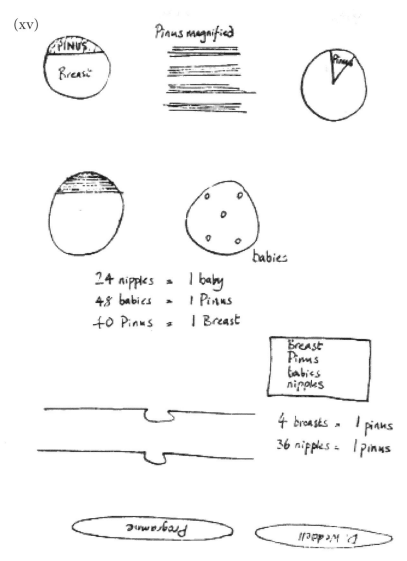

These were drawings rather like eyes and then there was what I took to be mirror writing, but also as if it was the eye at the bottom looking at things upside down, a kind of peeping-up-mummy's-bottom. He talked the whole session and was rather threatening towards the end, singing and swinging the rag around and trying to pull the chair away from me. When I had to hold his arm for a moment, he said, 'You shouldn't touch the penis', went out of the door muttering 'breast' and 'penis', but went up the corridor quietly, although there was a child there.

Friday, 5 February, 1965

Barry came in as I was going up the corridor and came down straight away. He began at once with a diagram on the left side of the wall (xvi). In this diagram there were what he labelled as two

(xvi)   (Front wall - 1)

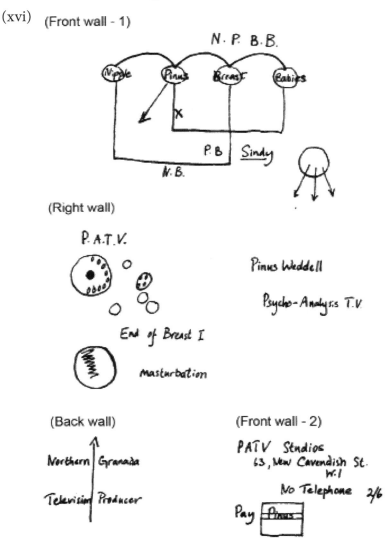

(Right wall)

(Back wall)

(Front wall - 2)

breasts with something like teeth and then perhaps a faeces-penis inside something like a spinal cord. Then there was 'psychoanalysis, language and television', and then he said, 'fault', writing on the wall 'masturbation'. Then something about 'the breast shouting and the penis stopped' and then 'end of breast 1'. He went back to the table and the papers and put lots of crosses on many pages while singing, but seemed to get back more in contact with me as I interpreted the retreat to omnipotence. Then he said something to the effect that it was hard to go on talking (in contrast to the previous day). Then there was 'Northern television, pay penis, James Bond, March 15th' and at the end of the session he attacked me so I had to hold him off, and he struck at my fingers and seemed to be wanting to touch me, which I linked with the problem of keeping his fingers away from his own genital. He went out but, opening the door twice, said something about 'breast-penis' and then went to wash his hands which had a lot of red chalk on them from writing on the wall.

Comment. The first drawing (for three months) of the nipple-penis-breast-babies all in circles and somewhat like teeth and gums, seemed to have some reference to the previous session when he had gone round the room saying that some places were penises, nipples, breasts and babies. It was very confusing, each object could change into the other. He had previously sung about 'Cindy, the doll you like to dress', as though it had some reference to the penis, the daddy, who dressed the mummy, who beautified the breast. In the 'psychoanalytic television' drawing, what appeared at first as a telephone dial, later seemed more to do with the breast that had places to put finger-penises in order to make it talk. Penis, finger and tongue seem interchangeable. In retrospect this was thought to have something to do with his silence.

Tuesday, 9 February 1965

With regard to the dentist, it looked as if he construed going to the dentist as a punishment for his oral sadism and that he was really expecting to be unable to do anything except suck as a result. Two days before that appointment, he said 'hello breast' as I went to the waiting room, and let the treatment door close on me, saying, 'Penis cut off in the breast'. I took up the problem of the unruly tongue, his use of language, his cutting off the meaning and the feeling from the action, distinguishing what was appropriate inside and outside the treatment room. Barry sat reading for more than half the session, occasionally singing, sometimes in a friendly even affectionate mood, which alternated with a frankly mocking, even obscene, manner.

He wrote on the wall 'Phil Silvers, Ill Silvers', then 'nothing wrong with the penis' and later, 'run rabbit, run'. At the end of the session Barry said, 'You are a woman analyst; your penis is too big', which seemed to be his recognition of the firm father inside the mother part of me, that could stand up to the sadism and the mocking.

Thursday, 11 February 1965

He was fifteen minutes late, rather pale, showed his teeth and said that the car had collapsed in Grays Inn Road, that he had come by taxi. I said that he was also telling me that he had been to the dentist and that I must distinguish between the collapse inside and the troubles outside. He said, 'No, sorry, the tyre was punctured.' Again he showed his teeth and said, 'Two fillings. No anaesthetic', but looked rather bleary-eyed and gazed at me in a squint-eyed way. He took the chalk and said, '3.40 to 4.10 today. 9.50 to 10.45 tomorrow'. I suggested that really he wanted to make up the lost time and he said 'Not today, have to go to coffee bar. Takes time to get there', and then shrieked and made a lot of 'ba-ba' noises.

But then he became rather subdued and perhaps a bit dysarthric, as if he had something in his mouth. His lips also seemed to be curling inwards but then he curled his top lip upwards and it became a sort of wolf smile. It was then as if he were an interviewer, asking lots of questions: 'Would you rather work with someone else and have other roles ?' he winked and said, 'Or would you work in a team in HMS Paradise. They all wanted to work in HMS Paradise.' Then 'PATV, the Show'. But this was written on the inside of the door of the chest of drawers. I questioned what he was not telling me? He wished that I should be able to see and know what was going on inside him. He said 'Next week's programme. Thursday, the Fugitive. Guest stars Rupert Davis, Ewen Solen', then 'HMS Paradise. Petty Officer Murdock becomes Lieutenant Eamonn Andrews, has his own show on ITV, also guest stars.' He went to the lavatory saying, 'If you want to know where I'm going, I shall be back after a few minutes.' On returning he took hold of my arm rather urgently and made me look at the inside of the door of the cupboard again and wiped the walls clean and left at 4.10. The office secretary came down to say that he had left ten shillings with her before he had come down to see me, and had taken it back as he left.

Going to the dentist was a very important occasion, of course; not only was he pleased that he had succeeded in staying in the dentist's chair and had some work done without an anaesthetic but also that he had come to the clinic by himself, the first time that this had occurred. Exactly four years later he was able to go by himself to a new dentist in a different hospital.

Friday, 12 February 1965

Barry was a few minutes late, whistling as he came down the corridor. He began to sing 'No, no, no' and took out his drawer and started to go through the paper. He put red crosses on some and I took up the distinction between internal and external damage. He hastened to reassure me that the car was standing still when the puncture occurred and then said, 'You're rubbish anyhow. I don't care'. I interpreted how much he did care, he had made the effort to get to the Clinic yesterday and today; though when I was not with him, a part of him said that I did not care and then that he did not either as he stamped and bit me ruthlessly in his mind. He was stamping on the chalk that he was dropping as he wrote on the walls: 'The Show, special guests Richard Caldicot, Frank Thornton, Robin Hunter, Ronald Rudd, Angus Lennie, Priscilla Morgan', and 'guests Rupert Davis, Ewen Solen, Victor Lucas'. Then these were reversed so the first became guests and the second series the special guests. He wrote, 'This is your life, says Eamonn Andrews to the paradise cast', 'those who have been in more than show' and 'this edition is introduced by Eamonn Andrews'. He wrote on another wall 'breast, penis, nipple, 2/6d, PA publications, 63 New Cavendish Street', then the price went down to l/3d, as I continued to interpret what double meaning I could detect. He said, 'Hello darling' and just before the end, blew into my eye and then reeled backwards, giving the impression of someone who was blind or drunk. He walked up the corridor singing quietly, about twelve minutes before the end of the session.

Monday, 15 February 1965

He was again late and was humming as he came down the corridor 'Hello darling' and 'She loves you'. He took the chalk out of the drawer and sat reading a weekly journal. Then he wrote on the wall 'Ring Collins if you want to know about Maigret. Fact or fiction, Agatha Christie', which I took up as giving me information about the deaths or murders of the weekend, that he wanted me to be on his wavelength, so that I should know what was happening. He cried 'cops' and, as the chalk broke, wrote 'Another neck broken', then 'PATV' and 'USATV, showtime with Danny Kaye, The Planemakers, the beloved of all Britons, Talk with Mike Tyman, BBC books, Danny Kaye'. There were variations on this theme, and he said that he was going at 4.10, 'USA Daniel Kalinski'. There was much breaking of chalk and as most of it was red or purple, the walls began to look bloodied again. I linked this with the war in Vietnam and the attacks on me, making me into a mummy whose body is the battle field where the children suffer and are killed by the bad 'U.S.' daddies at the weekend. I also linked it with his having been to the dentist and the bad teeth that were felt to have attacked and lacerated my nipple. He took up his papers at ten minutes before time and made 'bow-wow' noises. I was sitting in front of the door and did not move; he said, 'Why don't you get out of the way?', that he was going to meet his mother in the cafe, and 'It takes ten minutes to get there.' I pointed out that that was no reason to leave the session early. He looked absolutely furious and tried to force his way past me. I stood up and said I was not going to prevent him leaving but that we both knew that he was depriving the needy baby in himself by curtailing the session.

Tuesday, 16 February 1965

Barry was waiting, blew and spat at me and went to the lavatory on his way down, making faces at other people in the corridor and putting his hand to his genitals. He sat at the table reading horror books that he had brought, making quiet 'bow-wow' noises and small stampings with his feet. As I spoke about the end of the session the previous day, he made violent, agonizing cat-noises and then ambulance-sounds, which I linked to the moment of danger, the threat of violence and of an attack on me, reminding him of what had happened before and how nearly the wild animal part of him had taken control again. I suggested that the baby-part also had the temper tantrum when frustrated because the mummy-analyst did not impose her will on the wild-animal part.

He panted but this gradually subsided, though he went on looking through the books and then said 'PATV' and 'USATV, we'll continue till 4.20'; then 'New programme after Easter'. Then he made more accident noises, police sirens, hummed the 'Star-spangled banner' and 'Mine eyes have seen the glory', which I linked with his idea of my going away with my American husband and the danger of the war with me about the Easter holiday. He got up, took out some paper and wrote on it saying, 'Staying at home after all'. There seemed to be quite a lot of anxiety at this point in the session and he was picking his nose and ears and his finger was in his mouth, his back half-turned to me. As I went on talking, including saying that I was not yet sure what the Easter Holiday dates would be, he got up and came over, saying, 'For the whole session.' He wrote on the wall 'PATV 3, new programme, the world, United Kingdom', and he stayed until one minute before the end of the session, blowing at me as he went out, saying, 'Pig's mess'.

He seemed to have responded to the firmness of the expectation that he would stay to the end of the session, in a way that had become familiar whenever he felt confronted by the united parents (combined object).

Wednesday, 17 February 1965

Barry came in making kissing noises saying, 'Hello, pig's mess', and made more kissing sounds to a woman in the waiting-room, who took no notice. He gestured to go to the lavatory but then did not, slammed the treatment room door in my face as I went in behind him. Once in the room Barry wrote on the wall in column form, 'New programme, PATV, the world, the history of, puzzle, United Kingdom'. He came across the room and gave me a small piece of paper, Xmas card size, and then wrote on the wall 'Valentine, 1536, 154-0, French TV, very expensive, Arch de Triumph, Eiffel tower, Louvre, Notre Dame, President de Gaulle, General de Gaulle'. He again asked me about the holiday and this time I was able to give him the dates. He struck a comical attitude, pompous and mock-threatening, baring his teeth in a sort of monkey-face. 'Now what do you think you have gone and done?' he said, peering at me, then 'Don't let's waste time. We'll talk again at 4.10', as if he was the busy father who could not listen to complaints just then.

He wrote on the wall 'Switzerland' and then 'Basie' and then did a circle which was bisected so that there was a portion for D at the top and a sort of NE to NW half circle and then bisected it again in half, one with an F in it and one with an S in it. He said that he had forgotten the name of the French town and then something about beautiful passes, high mountains, as high as that wall, like blocks of flats, wrote 'Happy Show, New Show' and then changed it to 'Comedy, Danny Kaye, Phil Silvers, the Winter Brothers, Mark, Walter, Frank, more about it tomorrow'. At the end of the session he said it was clearing-up time and helped to clean the walls.

The reference to the Winter Brothers seemed to be his way of acknowledging that he felt persecuted in the holiday by the coldness of the frozen (Swiss mountain) breast. Some four years later he was at a stage when he could verbalize, 'I freeze you at the weekends – I put you in the freezer until Monday'.

Thursday, 18 February 1965

Barry came in as I walked up the corridor and said 'Hallo, Pig's breast'. As we walked down the corridor we met another child; Barry buried his head in his books in a way that suggested shyness rather than hostility. He sat at the table and as I talked he suddenly asked again about the holiday dates. When I repeated what I had told him the previous day he wiped a drip away from the end of his nose, stood up to get a handkerchief out of his pocket, blew his nose violently, and looked acutely miserable. He sat at the table with his head on his arm, quietly, and after a while he said, 'Saw ghost penis'. He then sat up and read for a bit but his nose was dripping and looked quite sore.

He then wrote on the wall and asked me if I remembered about the comedy playhouse yesterday, Comedy six. David Niven – father, Peter Sellers – Mike, Phil Silvers – Mark, Danny Kaye – John, Dick Van Dyke – Dick, Mary Tyler Moore – mother. Then he drew, saying something like '60 miles to the seaside … the winters used to go quickly in 1950 – not now'.

(xvii)

(a)

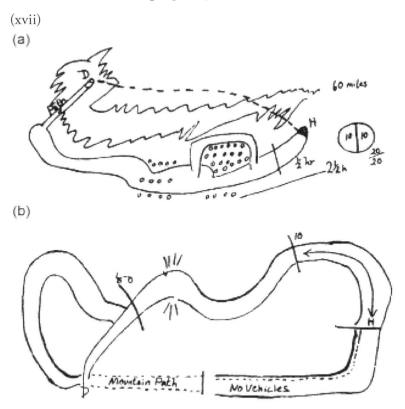

(b)

He drew another picture, several times muttering something about penis, talking in a very soft, hoarse voice, for he seemed to have a rather sore throat. Then 'Mystery, part 3, H equals house, D equals destination. The winters used to go a short cut, now it's a longer way around.' The first drawing (xvii) seemed to relate to his journey to the clinic, as on other occasions. The kind of ghost-like figure seemed to link with the ghost-penis. He had made some reference to the house where they had formerly lived as being all shut up, the boards up, as though it really contained something like the ghost of the dead babies, a haunted house. In the second drawing again there appeared to be references to the journey to and from the clinic, but I had the feeling that there was also something more to do with the analytic process, going up the mountain path, no vehicles, no masturbation. Perhaps there was a hint of a pregnancy, the eyes monitoring it as in the earlier 'shoe' drawing (xii). The lower drawing was thought to have something to do with the holiday and the experience of collapse. There certainly seemed to be some link with his getting a cold and what he said about winters and how he used to be able to go a short cut, now it's a longer way around.

I took this to be his acknowledgment that magic does not work any more. In fact in the countertransference it was a very moving session and reminded me of the second session of the analysis when he seemed to look so much like a little old man facing death. This time it was not so much facing death but really being miserable about the dead babies, the attacks on them, and about being left by the mummy in the infantile transference experience. In fact, he did not come the next day and I had a message to say that he had a bad cold. He was away two days in the next week as well.

Comment. In Phase 2 the 'castle' drawing of 12 November 1963 (xiv) had been taken to indicate the gradual conception of an internal world, an internal space within which phantasy could develop. In the sessions of Phase 3 just reported (4–18 February 1965) and particularly the drawings (xvii) of 18 February (eighteen months after drawing xiv), Barry seemed to be indicating his understanding that the route to the analyst (the clinic), embodied in a concrete fashion something of this state of mind during the journey. The double arrow seemed to be the coming and the going, indicating that he lost the newly acquired concepts as he got further away from the analyst, with some revival of memory as he returned.

From the beginning of treatment Barry had had a session on Friday mornings, the others being all at the same time in the afternoon. This had always been difficult for him; he would often be late and more tousled and out of contact than on other days. So this Thursday drawing, before an early Friday session, seemed to equate the holidays, the weekends, sleep and the difficulty of getting up, with being cold, snow, Switzerland, death and being out of contact. One had the impression from this that he appreciated that the only times he felt sane and in touch were during some analytic sessions, and that this experience and its loss was the core of a rhythmical process.

It seemed that one could postulate that the drawing indicated something like a unit of development; chaos, then as a result of interpretation, some splitting and idealization, projective identification, a little introjective identification just beginning, then renewed masturbatory attacks and the whole process to be repeated. At this time it seemed clear that Barry's mother carried the transference of the cafe-feeding mother while the analyst was mainly in the role of the toiletting mother. Compare, for instance, drawings (xvii) a-b with the earlier drawings (vii) a-b.

There also seemed to be the hint in this drawing that something terrible happened in his sleep, which could perhaps be linked with the little face, peeping out or drilling in and the devouring eyes of the early sessions. The nature of the sleep disturbance became clearer later in the analysis and will be outlined in the last section. It seems necessary to present the material in this massive way because, as a result of the continuous element of mystification in Barry's mode of communication, no single item or combination can carry much conviction for interpretation. Somehow, en masse, a grand, if vague, pattern can be discerned which then finds confirmation in later material.

Phase 4 (three-and-a-half to five years: 1965–68)

Synopsis. Crises of responsibility in relation to internal and external reality; problems of technique in the management of this phase are illustrated. Once established, there: was a diminution of aggression, destructiveness, obscenity and mocking, characterized by the cry, 'Now I know why I'm ugly!', with the emergence of affection, tolerance and optimism, in identification with the Mr Magoo-daddy.

The first crisis of responsibility had occurred in the third year of Barry's analysis, just before Whitsun, 1964. By this time he was nearly fifteen years old, and quite a young heavyweight. It became clear that if the analysis was to continue, Barry would have to be able to restrain the infantile aggression which still scratched, grabbed and kicked the analyst, whenever persecuted or frustrated. From the material already outlined, it seemed probable that he knew enough and could sufficiently distinguish the danger and the damage to himself as well as to the analyst, whenever it occurred.

This was explained to him, reminding him of what had already occurred in the analysis, emphasizing that the sixmonth to two-year-old baby could not do a great deal of physical damage in reality, though it might think that it could, but a two-year-old in the body of a fifteen-year-old could and might incapacitate the analyst for the next patient, which must not be allowed to occur.

It was characteristic of this child/young man, that he fought every inch of the way to discover if I really was determined not to be injured, while still being intent on interpreting what was happening between us as long as possible. It was then established between us that, whenever violence supervened, the session for that day would end, though we would recommence at the usual time on the next day and continue as long as there was no violence. The crisis came when I had to hold the treatment door closed after a particularly violent onslaught, while Barry kicked and pounded at the door, screaming and demanding to be let in. His mother stood by helplessly, then he kicked her, flew into the lavatory, kicked at the lavatory door, making a great noise, then burst into tears, and cried, 'Now I know why I am ugly'. He came out, kicked at the door again, turning to his mother saying pathetically, 'Why don't you do that?', the implication being that she should be firmer with him and more determined in her resistance to his violence and intrusion.

The sessions to be described now are taken from the week just before Whitsun, one year later, and three months after the 'mountain path' drawing. There had been something of a recurrence of violence and I had had to arrange that Barry's mother again bring him to the session and be on hand to take him home before the end of the session if necessary.

Wednesday, 26 May 1965

In this session his mother was in the waiting room and he made two loud snorting, farting noises at her as he came down the corridor to the treatment room. As he entered he said, 'Talking to the nipple. Have to talk to the nipple', leering and spitting at me. I interpreted the spoiling, his treating me as if I was a dirty nipple that enjoyed his dirty tongue. He sang sweetly but at the same time was using words in an obscene way, which was interpreted as the good music voice that is spoilt by the dirty tongue-words which dirty the beauty and food of the analytic breast.

Barry marched around, making lots of gassing noises and then began to write 'programme for today' on the door, walking backwards into me or making sudden lunges in my direction so that I had to quickly get out of his way. I warned him of the danger of this kind of attack on me. He danced around in a very provocative way and then collapsed on to me on the chair making pawing movements. I stood up and he began to write in purple on the wall something about 'third man' which I linked with the father-husband part of me and the holiday. He came towards me, collapsed into the chair, threw himself at me and I had to hold him off. I distinguished the fury of the little girl-part as well as that of the little boy-part towards the mummy when the daddy was felt to intrude and take me away for the holiday. He made for the door and rattled it, threatening to go out. He was warned that he knew that the treatment had to take place inside the room. He went out shouting, 'I want you, penis'. He went into the lavatory, came back singing very seductively, 'You are my girlfriend. Let me in', banging at the door. His mother came to the top of the corridor and he spat at her and shouted, 'Shut your face'. But eventually, grumbling, he said: 'Oh, all right', and went up to her.

In retrospect I thought the session was under the influence of the Cassius Clay–Sonny Liston heavyweight fight that had taken place the night before. He had tended to behave like a younger version of Cassius Clay on other occasions.

Thursday, 27 May 1965

He was whistling as he came down and called out, 'Hello penis', but looked more subdued. He sat at the table reading and singing 'penis and nipple'. I took this up as taking the meaning out of experiences concerned with love and beauty. I suggested that he was creating an ugly caricature of the analytic parents' love-making and had done the same yesterday, raising the question of a link to the Clay–Liston fight. My emphasis was on his misuse of words for body-parts, and I did this every time he started to use these words in such a manner. Immediately there was a change and eventually it came round to his singing 'oranges and lemons, just slipping in the word penis, or breast or nipple, in a way more like slips of the tongue. At the same time he was poking his tongue out, but eventually he sang   correctly, the last line being taken as 'big bell of bow, bow, bow', in a lugubrious voice. He got up and then wrote 'programme for today'. It was written on the door, then wiped out and written on the wall: 'News. Survival, Rawhide, Richard Lionhearted' . It was underlined and written several times, then 'Dr. Kildare, Raymond Massy' then 'Romeo'.

A dangerous situation now seemed to occur again with farts and gassing sounds, but this seemed to be controlled by my talking and a 'pardon' was slipped in as he walked in front of me. I distinguished the different dangers of the inside and outside world and the problem of the Hitler-gassing-part linked with the weekend. He crossed to the other wall and wrote in blue 'this week, revived, next week'. I said that his mother would continue to bring him to the session until after Whitsun. He then wrote 'new series' and drew a circle (xviii) which seemed to have something like an eye in it but as a little 'c' in the centre. He then drew a smaller circle with a little 'u' in the centre so that the two together looked like eyes, one looking aside and the other looking down. He wrote 'D W T V travel' then in large letters 'north, London east, south', with E and W to the left and right, but all very far apart, saying 'cold at the weekend', which I took up in terms of his anger with me, turning cold towards me when I was

(xviii)

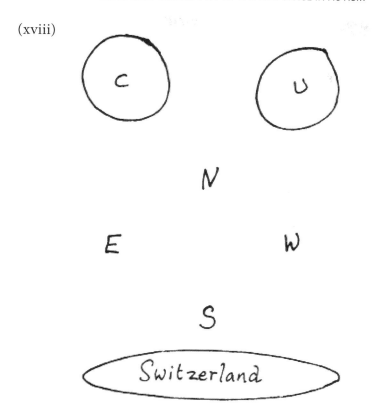

felt to turn him out, when he felt that I would not see him. He said, 'Snow', but then altered the north and south so that they were closer together. He wrote 'new travel film with Douglas J', and then wrote 'Switzerland', and said something about difficulty in getting through, 'Have to be postponed until tomorrow', then wrote 'Switzerland' in the middle of an elliptical figure, and departed from that session quietly.

Friday, 28 May 1965

Barry was late and a long while coming down to the treatment room, having a noisy altercation with his mother, shouting down the corridor at me, 'I'm coming, penis'. There were children in the waiting-room and his mother was protesting and he seemed to be trying to show her up as quite helpless. He walked out into the corridor saying he was 'not going to see Miss Weddell', and she looked down the corridor at me despairingly. Eventually he came down shouting 'nipple, penis' at me. I took up the problem of the language again, the tongue that ran away with him, that would be obscene and mocking toward a good relationship; also the problem of his trying to shock the other children, trying to drive them away.

He wrote on the wall 'psychoanalytic television', and then on another wall 'take the nipple into the breast, add the penis and the masturbation'. Then 'line up', underneath that 'Psychoanalytic television', then as a column: 6-8 penus —6.30 breast —7.00 take your penis—7.30 masturbation—8.00 ice skating—8.30 masturbation - Tame.

On the door in column fashion: '5.55 News—6.05 Penis—P P T V—6.30 take your penis. —P.P. —7.00 Music P.A. —7.15 Breast P.P. —7.30 masturbation P.N. —8.45 ice skating A T V — 8.15 Ward 10 A T V —8.45 A T V —9.00 News I T V. 9.10 World in Action—9.40 Red Cap—10.35 Cinema.'

On the other wall again in columns: 'F S C—P.A. B B C 4— D W T V. Parallel to that: F S C—P A T V—P B T V—P P T V—P M T V—P N T V', with two strokes leading to 'F S C – 2' and one stroke leading to 'D W T V'.

Then there was another version of 'P A T V' in hieroglyphics which I could not understand but which ended in R S G L and underneath that 4 Y P which I thought was a mix-up with the registration numbers of my car and its predecessor. Again a column headed 'F S C—5.45 News—5.55 Richard the Lionheart—Comedy Hour—Music—Not Time for Sergeants—News— Red Cap—Burke's Law— Car 54—Freud's Hour—News—Close Down.'

All this time he had been very mocking and obscene, as I continued to talk and to interpret to him the nature of the attacks and the danger. When we got to Burke's Law we seemed to be getting to a point in which the toiletting nature of the relationship was beginning to give relief. When we came to Freud's Hour I thought this probably was the nodal point of the session with the acknowledgment of the Freud-daddy nipple. He wrote 'Freud's Hour' on another wall and underneath this 'The Human Jungle' and underneath that 'Penis, nipple, masturbation, breast'. And then parallel with it 'Comedy Hour. HMS Paradise. The

Lynne Show'. Underneath that 'Red Cap. John Shaw. A Sergeant John Man' and then more programmes this time with the 'Burke's Law' taken out but put back later on.

I continued to talk of the importance of keeping the Freud's Hour, the analytic hour, the time for sorting out what goes wrong in the jungle of his unconscious, the relics of which were felt to be in the faeces. Then of the penis, nipple, breast and babies attacked in the masturbation, by the mocking part of him that would make a comedy of the analyst-parents when they were felt to be having intercourse in the state of mind equated with paradise. All of this was linked with the difficulty of the weekend for him. He clawed and scratched towards me as he left but without actually touching me.

Monday, 31 May 1965

There was some delay in coming down and he said, 'Hello penis' in a rather provocative manner, singing 'penis and breast'. My continued interpreting seemed to result in an alteration in his feeling and eventually he was humming 'Land of hope and glory'. He then read comics for some minutes and continued to sing, making occasional references in a rather obscene mechanical way to nipple, penis, breast, which I interpreted on each occasion in a manner already indicated. He got up and wrote 'P.A.T.V.' on the door and 'programme and F S C' and 'his own TV2' on the wall and then there were all kinds of alterations in these programmes but the principal ones seemed to be the introduction of Mr. Magoo. There were also alterations to 'No Hiding Place' which was eventually changed to 'Panorama' and 'Bewitched' and 'Perry Mason'. Much farting, not just gassing noises, and at one point after he had passed me leaving a smell, said 'I apologise, nothing to do with analysis. Upset tummy'. I questioned whether he had been making a stink with his mother at the weekend because he was angry with me and whether he had been eating food he knew was liable to upset him (linked with an earlier session in which he said he had been eating too much cheese). I took up the gassing attacks on the children at the clinic, as my babies, and he said, 'Shut up'. I interpreted that he had tried to shut me up inside him over the weekend and treated me as though I was to be in his concentration camp bottom, attacked with every form of torment.

Barry began to drum a military rhythm on the table, but it eventually became an SOS which I interpreted as a need for help at the weekend, his recognition of this and the problem of having to wait when he felt identified with the baby and mother who might both die from his gassing attacks. There were more changes in the programme and he said, 'Apologising for little notice', which at the time I thought might be linked with the Queen's child who had suddenly gone into hospital at the weekend for an ear operation. He lay across the table as if he were going to die, which I interpreted as his insistence that he was my analysis Royal baby going to die, poisoned from within by farts. When I reminded him of the long weekend at Whitsun, he got up and wrote 'calculated risk'. I distinguished the kind of risks I had to take, the risks there were in the outside world and the problem of protecting the mummy inside him; that, when he could do this, all the outside world risks became less threatening. He spent the last part of the session in provocativeness and threats of attacks with kicks, scratching and throwing things at me, but in the end he stayed the full time.

Tuesday, I June 1965

He was halfway down the corridor by himself and noisy as he came in, knowing that he was expected to wait until I was ready for him. I showed him at this point why it was not possible to take him to my private consulting room for treatment and that this would not be possible until he, the big boy part of him, could control his violence. He continued to be very noisy and singing 'penis and breast' at intervals, but was obviously listening to what I was saying, at the same time writing out 'programmes' all over the walls. He wiped some off, which was unusual, but made many alterations. Mr Magoo came in again; Mike Richards, Cannon Ball, Necklace, Survival. Again there was much gassing and he flung the wet rag around and wiped it around the top of the table and then over his face.

Barry then wrote on the table 'This is your life. Repeat'. I talked about his messing me up and squeezing the last drop out of me until I was exhausted and worn out (this being a reference to the state I had been left in after the previous session, which had not seemed outwardly extraordinary, but which nevertheless left me feeling unusually exhausted). He tore the rag to pieces and used bits of paper to wipe the wall and then used paper to make telescopes which I linked with his peeping inside me to see the damage. During this session I insistently tried not to use any of the words he defamed and took up each time how he was taking the meaning out of emotional experiences when he used 'penis' or 'breast' in such a manner. He wrote 'You must be punished' and repeated it in a very mechanical Dalek-like voice, but left singing 'not so much a programme, more a way of life'. There was less mess on the walls but more mess on the floor.

Wednesday, 2 June 1965

Barry was noisy, rude and attacking his mother at the top of the corridor. When he came down I spoke strongly of the danger to the analysis of that kind of behaviour and of his mocking and defiant, denigrating tongue. I talked standing with my back to the door, with my 'policeman hand' up, as he was very threatening. Then he came towards me in a less threatening manner and looked at my hand in a way that made me think he was treating it as if it were a crystal ball. I took up his wish to see into me, see what was going on inside my mind. He continued to dodge backwards and forwards but eventually retreated and threw the soap at me. Then on the wall he drew (xix) a number of pictures (the first again for six months). These pictures are illustrated, but to describe them briefly: there was a picture called 'Miss Weddell inside world' and my hair was made very tall with something like a penis inside it and with two horns sticking out of it. (Earlier in the analysis he had referred to me as Devil). On another wall he drew something like a Union Jack, a flag with 'Mr Magoo' written on it and 'The Wedding Ceremony' and called it 'People in Love'. While he was doing this he said that I 'had given him the word penis'. I reminded him of the first session when he had been scratching himself but agreed that what I had said seemed to have been experienced as if I had put a penis into his mouth rather than a nipple. He washed out the rag and washed his hands and sang for a while.

(xix)

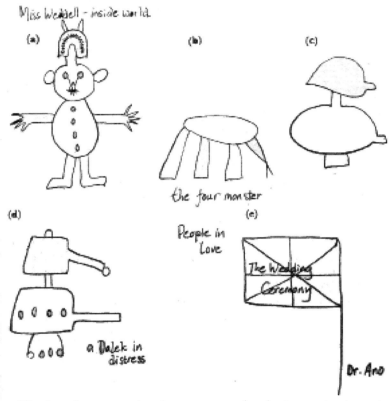

He then began to sing in a very tender, loving voice in quite a poetic manner, 'Mr Magoo went for a walk one night in the dark, in the dark. To his surprise he met a young woman. He met a young woman to his surprise, surprise. He suddenly felt that he was in love, that he was in love, a lover. It was so long, so late. Could it really be that he was in love, a lover at last?' He then talked in quite a different voice for a few minutes, something about 'Town and Around, and 'Pardon the Expression' and 'Mr Ed'. But he then smeared green chalk on his shoes, on the floor and on the rug before he left. It is probably important that Mr Magoo has very defective vision and compensatory optimism.

This was an extremely moving session, the first time that something came across as affection, wonder, mystery and enlightenment. It seemed likely that his identification of him self with a Magoo-daddy heralded a curtailment of intensive voyeurism into the breast and the beginnings of gratitude to it.

Comment. In this section, sessions have been described to illustrate the developing of many crucial concepts in the infantile transference, concepts of internal space, the geography of phantasy; the conception of roles, of a mental pathway, of a centre of existence, of a time/space relationship, of cold and warmth, of combined parents, of damage and of love. All are further elaborations of what seemed to have begun to be established in the previous phase though perhaps the developing capacity for co-operation and affection was the most hopeful for the ultimate outcome of the analysis.

Fifth year of analysis (1968)

Synopsis. Barry goes to school and begins to report dreams that confirm and illuminate earlier material and clarify earlier interpretations. Various meanings of sleep emerge and the struggle over the concept of work begins.

It was possible for Barry to be brought to the analyst's private consulting room, and begin to lie on the couch at four years of treatment (when age fifteen and a half). Plans were made for him to attend a special school at the beginning of the next academic year. This idea became known between us as P.A.C. (Psychoanalytic conspiracy). In Barry's mind all the psychoanalysts were involved and felt to be forcing him out of the gorilla-like way of life, 'even though he could now use the toilet and the shower', his words on leaving the clinic.

On the day that Barry went to school for the first time, he entered the consulting room in a well-held-together manner, with a briefcase under his arm; quite a different picture from that of the loose-limbed fat boy of the previous months. My feeling was that some identification with a working-daddy was occurring. He collapsed on to the couch and slept for most of the session.

There had been brief uneasy moments of sleep earlier in the analysis, but this time it was different. As he lay there, slightly flushed, something of a pink and white angel-baby seemed to emerge from out of his grossness. My impression was of a birth situation being re-enacted, a 'mother and baby doing well' kind of picture, with relief all round: quite a moving experience in the counter-transference.

Sleep in the session continued for some months. On the first occasion only did it appear to be restful sleep, for some time subsequently it was very disturbed. Barry then began to report his night dreams: he had only presented two or three previously, on each occasion related to my death.

The following is a dream reported in a mid-week session and quoted in part, at the beginning of the paper: *He had to go to a laboratory. There was a computer there, into which he had to feed the analyst's name and address. Lots of people were there, they each had earphones and a receiver. Six months later, he came back and each had a box in front of him. When he looked inside his own box, there was an effigy of himself, a kind of death mask, a horrible monster, with four eyes, noses and mouths, ten legs and arms.* As Barry told me the dream, his voice trailed off and he slept.

This dream is, I think, reminiscent of much that I have already outlined, and recalled to me many sessions similar in material. Thus it will not be difficult for readers to share something of my experience of wonder, at the clarity wrought by the analytic process. The dream could be interpreted with fair conviction that it was my laboratory and his lavatory; that the computer, the toilet-breast-mummy, was also a feeding-breast-mind, which not only receives his abusive names but could also show him the truth about himself gradually, in time, when he was able to bear it, in retrospect, having already made some progress.

The existence of other children at the clinic was acknowledged in the dream. It had been important to Barry at the beginning of analysis that they were protected from his intrusive, terrorizing impulses, as he had been from their retaliations, in contrast to the situation of his internal world, where the mother appeared to be constantly attacked, aborted, and, with her children, mutilated or murdered. In this sense, the analyst had been experienced as a strong enough object, to withstand his annihilating attacks, while continuing to hold him, contain him, not drop him down the lavatory as a faeces-baby.

The six months later, in the dream, was in reality more like four years, an indication of Barry's difficulty in relation to time. Clearly, however, he could at that point understand something of the effigy, monster part of himself and the relationship with his eight octopus fingers and ten arms and legs. He could face the horror of such a picture of himself rather than impose it on others by aggressive behaviour, as at the beginning of analysis.

For the remainder of the session, during the time that Barry was apparently asleep, I talked aloud on these themes. When I woke him just before it was time, he said 'Remarkable', looking at me intently, 'and it happens when I take a nap', giving me a beatific smile as he left.

The next day, Barry again reported a dream in which *he was in a big car; then found that he was sitting in a coffin* (an association to President Kennedy's death). *He called to his friend to come and help him out and to tell him why he was there. His friend helped him out but when he wanted a nap he got in again and pulled down the lid. Then he heard beautiful music, and when he looked up, everything was different.*

This dream was interpreted in relation to the end of the session of the previous day, for it seemed to confirm that, for Barry, going to sleep (taking a nap) was equated with getting into a coffin (closing his eyes — pulling the lid down). It also seemed clear that it was the analyses voice, as his mother's voice in the past, that rescued him and brought about the recognition of life and beauty (everything different).

Two weeks later, Barry described another dream. *He had made a safe landing on the moon.* This was interpreted at the time, as the patient being able to feel well held and protected, by a moon-breast, able to sleep in a lively way, very different from getting-into-the-coffin kind of sleep.

After another four weeks' work, mostly in relation to masturbatory phantasies, concerned with slipping into projective identification with the father's penis (dreams of going to the moon in a rocket), there was another important change. This time Barry dreamed that *he landed on the moon; the Emperor came and said that it was his territory, but he could stay there for a time.* This seemed clearly enough to be Barry's acknowledgment that he had internal combined objects (breast-moon and emperor-nipple) who had the capacity for speech and could differentiate situations for him in a helpful way (introjective identification).

The possibility of healthy curiosity and co-operation seemed to be established. It seemed strongly suggested by this sequence of dreams that action (behaviour, drawings and use of language} of the previous five years or so, could now be better contained and transformed from dream-thoughts to verbal communications, implying an improved differentiation between internal and external reality. This was confirmed outside the analysis in that Barry was able at that time to tolerate the discipline of an understanding school environment and seemed to be making up for lost educational time.

Comment. In retrospect, one can see how easily the computer of the first dream could have originally been equated with Barry's bottom, to which his eight octopus fingers were addicted. In that sense, his bottom would have been a satisfactory substitute for a breast, which was experienced as a permeable, defenceless object: in Bion's terms, a container lacking sensitivity or capacity for reverie; in Bick's terms, without sufficient skin to function as a boundary.

After a period of years (not of weeks as in the dream}, the breast was recognized by Barry as a box-container (linked with his TV addiction), a mirror-breast that could reflect back to the baby pictures of himself in a way that made the pain of seeing himself as an effigy, as a greedy monster, a parasite and an addict, tolerable for him.

The death mask could also be thought of as the equivalent of Bion's idea of 'nameless dread' and of the infant's fears of his dying. From the subsequent dream of being in a coffin, sleep and death were seen to be equated, throwing light on one of the meanings of sleep in the sessions. 'Sitting in the coffin' strongly suggests falling into the dead breast, linked with the fear of being found to be a faeces-baby who is allowed to throw himself away in the toilet.

In the dream, at that point in time, the patient was able to 'call for help', to be pulled out of his state of projective identification. In the dream, Barry's friend (the analyst-nipple), helps him out. The next time he gets into the coffin-sleep (in the session}, as he awakens he looks up at the nipple, not down to the bottom, with the result that 'everything is different'.

'Looking up' and 'everything different' can then be related to the next dream of the moon breast on which Barry makes a safe landing and, importantly, does not get inside. He can sleep with it, not in it. Again it would seem to be the object's, the breast's, capacity to support the baby and to resist intrusions, invasive projective identifications, that makes such a change possible (Money-Kyrle) .

In the next dream, we see a link with all the work of the analysis, resulting in policemen-guardsmen-penises being allowed to protect the Queen-mother-breast-analyst. In the dream, the Emperor-nipple is felt to have the strength, integrity (not subverted by masturbatory intrusions) to be able to ration time and space for the baby, and thus there seems to be the recognition of a benevolent combined-object.

In sequence this followed Barry's conceptualization of an object that can accept the baby's distress about where it is, what it is doing, understand it and return that knowledge to the baby in a manner that gives relief, allowing (in Bion's terms) a 'growth stimulating part of the personality' to develop. The struggle over the use of time continued for several months. Sleeping in the session was then seen as primarily a defence against oedipal jealousy, particularly before and after weekends. It also emerged as a defence in relation to conflict with me as an external object, about the nature of analytic work and of co-operation. Staying awake meant feeling the pain; 'I cut off your head and your feet', as Barry said in relation to use of time in the session when arriving late and leaving early. This could also be linked with his earlier statement, 'I cut you up and stick you back all over the place', to illustrate how he came to be out of touch with time. Slowly, as introjective identification proceeded, a transformation occurred. From out of the falling asleep, of the parasitic ensconcement within the object, working for longer periods in the session became possible.

Externally, he was able to walk into the consulting room in a clearly 'well held together' manner, very different from the 'Baboon' of the early months of the analysis. But he still tended to collapse on to the couch in an elephantine way (elbows and knees). Eventually this became known as 'elephantiasis'.

By the seventh year of analysis (1969), something of the struggle over work, and the changing internal picture, was illustrated in a dream. *Barry was in a train, with lots of rooms in it, for families. There were corridors, so you could walk about, and places for cars. When they came to a difficult hilly part, a diesel engine wasput on; much better for pulling up hills.* Something of the nature of the analytic work seemed to have been recognized, and an internal part-object that had the capacity for hard work appeared to have been introjected. It strongly suggests the configurations of drawings xiv (b) and xvii (b) combined.

Subsequently, as healthy projective and introjective identification proceeded (the putting in and taking out, as in the computer dream), Barry began to be able to distinguish a healthier, more adult part of himself and could verbalize, 'I bring my baby part to you'. He could make contact in the session without being the baby. It then became possible for him to begin to carry out parental functions towards the baby-self. He could cook, clean his room. He could stay in the house alone and was working in the holidays. Some inroads had been made into the depressive position and Barry was able to distinguish 'what matters is, which eye you use to view people, the box machine eye or the human eye' (Bion's reversible perspective?). His parasitism was still in evidence, and his reluctance to work, and wish to remain dependent on his family, but progress continued in the analysis.

Summary of theoretical formulations

Detailed clinical material had been given in sequence that appears to the writer to illustrate some aspects of the development of an internal world in a boy, recovered from an autistic state but with a gross psychotic character development.

The thesis of this paper in so far as it is understood in relation to the material presented, has been that for Barry an object to be available for helpful projective identification of a part in distress, relieving that part, and returning it to the self for integration

(Bion), has to be an object sufficiently strong and resilient to be able to withstand invasive projective identification (Bick) and the parasitic ensconcement of that part, within the object (Meltzer).

For Barry, in the first phase of analysis, the turning point seemed to occur with the recognition of the analyst as an object, that could be vulnerable but could recover, that had a skin that could be damaged but could heal, under the bandage, between sessions. In Barry's mind, wounds became orifices. This phase was followed by the development of the phantasy of internal policemen-doctor-penises that restored and protected the analyst, giving rise to the conception of an internal world containing spaces, and of objects with spaces within. This gradually became equated with an internal family with roles, relationships, functions and need for privacy.

Material from Barry's second and third phases as described seemed to illustrate something of how intrusive projective identification (violent destructive phantasies and omnipotent voyeurism) changed to more helpful projective identifications (Canadian Mounted Police, doctors as TV stars, etc.}, with gathering evidence of healthier curiosity (Bion's growth stimulating part of the personality). As introjective identification began to occur, then benevolence and affection could impinge on aggression.

Barry's transformation from the ugly-gorilla-effigy-monster through to a young man who could hold himself erect, act purposefully and on occasions appear quite personable, seems to confirm the impression of the material, that this improvement depended on the strength, resilience and integrity of internal objects, through introjective identification.

Later, through his dreams, we could understand that the analyst's computer-mind was equated with a toiletting-breast, an object, a container, into which he felt he could expel his unwanted, painful, threatening experiences. It was equated with the coffin-breast, an object that should relieve the baby of its fear of dying (Klein, Bion} and its dead objects. Such an object seems to become equated by the baby with its own bottom (Meltzer) which is thus the defenceless, permeable object confused with a helpless breast, an object inside of which the baby feels it can ensconce itself or parts of itself as a parasite (Meltzer).

When these parts were well enough, firmly enough contained (Bick) then the toiletting-breast became also the mirror-box breast, that showed the baby pictures of itself and what it had been doing, that can be equated with the breast as an object that can denude an experience of pain (Bion), an object that has a space for receiving the baby's experiences and the capacity for returning them to the baby for healthier development (Klein, Bick). From Barry's material, the coffin-breast could then become the moon-breast (i.e. after it was explained to Barry how he had got into the coffin), and he was helped out of his projective identification, so that introjective identification could begin with an undamaged object. The differentiation was then established between getting in, putting a part in (going to the moon in a rocket), and taking back, separation (landing on the moon for a short while).

Once the containing function of the breast and its availability for helpful projective identification was established, together with the concept of an internal world, containing spaces, there seemed to be a lessening of projective identification, and with that introjective identification with undamaged objects began to occur. This brought with it admiration and respect for personal qualities (the emperor, rationing time and space, the diesel engine, pulling up hill), as a bulwark against persecution by damaged objects which were so confused with bad objects and bad parts of the self.

This development seems in line with Bick's idea of the skin functioning as a boundary, with Bion's of a holding, containing, capable-of-reverie object and with Bick's thesis that until such an object can be introjected, the phantasy of internal and external space is impaired. It also seems to confirm her view, that in the absence of such introjection, projective identification continues unabated, giving rise to difficulties in healthy development, illustrated by Bick in relation to objects 'without a skin', and Meltzer in the 'parasitic ensconcement of part of the self within an object'.

CHAPTER SIX

The residual autistic condition and its effect upon learning – Piffie[1]

Shirley Hoxter

The main concern of this chapter will be to study some factors which appear to have impeded or enhanced one particular boy's capacity for growth. Christopher, usually known as 'Piffie', commenced psychotherapy with me at the age of three and a quarter years. He attended four times weekly for the most part, until he was eight and a quarter, when treatment was terminated. Two and a half years later his therapy was recommenced and, from eleven until fourteen (his age at the time of writing) he has attended once weekly.

The periods of psychotherapy to be discussed mainly concern the residual effects of an autistic state. Piffie was probably beginning to emerge from this state before he commenced psychotherapy and he shed its more blatant manifestations within the first year of therapy. Nevertheless traces of former autistic features may still be discerned and they continue to have a constricting effect upon his development.

---

1   First published in the *Journal of Child Psychotherapy,* 3(2): 21–39, 1972.

Early history and background

Christopher is the youngest of three children. At the time of his birth, by caesarian section, his mother was very anxious, having from her previous experiences reason to fear that he might die. In fact he was a healthy, but a very passive baby, sleeping a great deal and never grasping the nipple or bottle teat sufficiently strongly to suck properly. Milk had to be practically poured into him.

At about two and a half a medical friend drew his parents' attention to his condition. At that time his meaningful contact and response to people and things around him was so meagre that the possibilities of his being deaf or mentally defective were investigated. At the time of his referral to me at three and a quarter his development was immature in every respect except that of motor development. He could say a few single words, but rarely did so. Those of his activities which did not seem to be purposeless restlessness consisted mainly of putting things in and out of boxes. He was said to show no enjoyment in play or zest for life. He often spent long periods gazing into space apparently oblivious to his surroundings; this was especially apparent at times of major changes such as a seaside holiday. He was highly sensitive, however, to minor changes, particularly any which impinged upon one of his many routines. (He was said to have a routine for everything.) He was extremely demanding and, when frustrated, he readily collapsed into prolonged screaming attacks. His terror and fury were particularly marked when being taken out of the house or out of the push-chair or when being put into new clothes. He had severe feeding and sleeping difficulties but was clean and dry by day. He had a small bald patch on the top of his head due to constant hair tugging.

Piffie's mother was an exceedingly vulnerable and over anxious person. She was very concerned for him but was constantly harassed, guilty, feeling she must give in to him about everything. There were many occasions to observe that when Piffie communicated his anxieties to his mother, she responded by rushing her own anxieties into him. Fortunately, however, it was possible to arrange for mother to have sessions with a psychiatric social worker who has greatly helped her.

Father has given much support both to his wife and to the maintenance of the treatment situation. However, he, too, frequently expressed severe lack of self-confidence. Piffie's condition at referral may be summed up in his mother's words: 'He seems afraid of life.'

Educational history

I will now give a summary of his subsequent history with particular reference to his education. He was tested at the age of ten and obtained 1.Q. 126. Between the ages of four and five years Piffie's understanding and use of words reached a level at least normal for his age, although his speech was indistinct. By five he had the full range of skills which one would expect of an intelligent pre-school child. His social and emotional difficulties, however, continued to be severe and it was necessary to delay his entry into school for a further year. Shortly before his sixth birthday he commenced attending an ordinary preparatory school, at first attending part-time only in a class of children who were younger than himself. He soon moved up to join his own age-group and shortly before he was seven went to a conventional private preparatory school where he was rapidly placed ahead of his age-group. At thirteen he obtained a scholarship to a highly selective senior school.

Until he was approaching twelve years of age school attendance was a source of severe suffering for him. Leaving his mother and home, and having to endure the torments of others boys of whom he was terrified, caused him agonies. He was frequently near to school refusal especially at times of changing class or teacher. He was able to endure school largely by utilizing a pathological process which enabled him to keep school and home life in rigidly separated compartments. His drive towards intellectual achievement was undoubtedly reinforced by flight from social life in school but it would be an over-simplification to regard this as a major factor.

The scholarship he obtained suggests a success story so far as scholastic achievement is concerned. But a closer knowledge of Piffie reveals the deceptive nature of these achievements and leads to fuller recognition of the ways in which his apparent progress in therapy has been deceptive in the past. He achieved an impressive accumulation of knowledge but made relatively little educational progress of a nature which could lead to an enhancement of comprehension or creativity.

He changed from functioning as a mental defective to functioning as a pedant. Yet some essentials of his learning difficulties hardly altered. These particularly concern his obsessional mechanisms and will form the main theme of the chapter.

The early stages of psychotherapy

My first impressions of Piffie at age three and a half years were of an attractive child, small for his age but compact and chubby, who showed a baffling degree of self-composure and lack of anxiety. In the first session he showed no reaction when his mother left the room. He spent much of his time examining building blocks and little toys, lining them up, grouping them in a variety of arrangements and then carefully packing them away in boxes. He glanced at me twice and his first use of me was to get me to hold two blocks which had fallen down. During the first weeks this was to be one of his most frequently repeated activities. It was apparent that the toys (little animals, houses, cars etc.) had almost no representational value to him, they were largely undifferentiated bits and pieces of himself and his objects. Unlike some more severely autistic children he did not discharge these bits all around him with the effect of producing in the room a state of chaos which both reflects the inner state and obliterates the distinction between self and non-self. Instead Piffie showed a persevering need to control bits and to impose upon them his own private sense of order in which location and the use of containers, such as boxes, played an important part. In the following sessions he showed anxiety and fury about things which fell on the floor and would not conform to his systems. He then began to use my lap in a way somewhat differentiated from the boxes as a place for things which were fallen, muddled or otherwise troublesome. This often led to exploring the contents of my lap, and retrieving from it things which were then apparently more meaningful to him. For when he took them from my lap he became increasingly able to name them appropriately and from this beginning his use of speech steadily increased.

I will give some examples from the third and fourth week of therapy. First he wanted to make sure that all his toys were as he had left them before the weekend. They were in a box, which was in another box, which was in a third box which was in a drawer. He particularly wanted to find the toy lioness which, using one of his rare words, he called Gigi after the cat at home. After a while he loaded all the toys into my lap. He then searched for Gigi and found her with pleasure and repeated this play of losing Gigi under the mass of toys and finding her again. My interpretation included that he wanted me to be a mummy who could safely hold all his things inside me; that Gigi (representing I think the cuddly, comforting aspects of the maternal object he had lost over the weekend) kept getting lost and mixed up with all the plop plops and other things which he felt he had put into me and that, when I held these, he felt he could look into me and find the good parts again. After this he took up and named a number of other toys, rabbits, windows on a house and a 'daddy horse'.

In a session of the fourth week he discarded some blocks and threw them into my lap with some violence. He tried to build with the remaining blocks and it was clear that their yellow and blue colouring played an important part in his arrangement. He was never satisfied with his structure and it kept falling down; he became somewhat desperate, crying a little, clenching his teeth and looking furiously at me. At last he took the fallen pieces, placed them in my lap and tried to build there. I interpreted his need for me as a mother who could receive his attacks and the fragments of himself. To make my interpretation clearer to him I showed how the yellow and blue blocks stood for himself, wearing a yellow jumper and blue shorts. He was delighted at this and immediately went to get some red blocks which he placed on his red shoes, showing me how they matched. For him this was a moment of real insight and relief. He then took a little tower with a red top and held it near his penis. Following this, with the blocks still in my lap, he successfully put together a construction with red blocks as his shoes at the base, then blue blocks for his shorts and the yellow ones for his jumper.

This way of putting the pieces of himself together and achieving a more coherent image of himself and his body represented elementary but important steps towards a sense of identity. By putting parts of his self into me as a containing mother he began to discover a way of coping with his feelings of being in pieces and to find himself. For a while after this he began most sessions by finding the appropriate blocks to match the colouring of his clothing and of mine. He now had a play language with which to express and, as it were, to think out his problems. In this way he could communicate and work upon what I then understood to be the vicissitudes of integration, disintegration, loss or damage to parts which he felt us both to undergo. The parts of his own body and of mine could be better differentiated and there could be more distinction between what was himself and what was someone or something else.

Discussion

It is typical of the history of Piffie and his psychotherapy that developments such as those just described are deceptive. Retrospectively I continue to consider that these advances had the meaning and value described. But only too often his systematic perseverance over a problem has become perseveration and the step forward is found to have been a step leading into a culde-sac. I would now consider that this material also referred to the most stubborn aspects of his psychopathology, those concerning his primitive obsessional mechanisms. In this example placing the blocks together to represent himself appeared to be a communication about the integration of an object which had been split into fragments. I would now consider it as a precise and literal statement concerning the assemblage of an object which had been segmented into portions. Such an object can, just like the building blocks, be assembled, segmented again and then reassembled in endless permutations, but it cannot undergo the healing process of reparation or the growth process of integration.

When we talk of an object as having been split we usually have in mind that it has been divided along lines of emotional experience. Different emotional experiences and the sources to which they are attributed are kept apart. In normal early splitting the maternal object is divided: one part is idealized and felt to be the source of all that is gratifying and this is distanced from another part which is experienced as persecutory. An object which has been segmented or dismantled (Meltzer) is an object which has been reduced to small simplified portions, usually according to segments of sensory experience, rather than split upon lines of emotional and potentially mental experience. For example, the autistic child may have one maternal object which has a taste, another which has a smell, a sight, a sound and so on. Similarly he will have a tasting self, a seeing self, a hearing self, etc. These segments of object may then be kept apart and one by one omnipotently controlled. Or, for example, the mother who can be heard and the self who can hear may be discarded in favour of an inanimate object equated with a part of mother who/which can be held in the hand and manipulated at will.

This view of autism is one which places major emphasis upon the employment of primitive forms of obsessional mechanisms. It gives a fresh perspective to the consideration of the autistic child's malfunctioning perceptual system, his lack of mentation and his stereotyped behaviour.

Piffie frequently experienced his object and himself as segmented but his dissections followed rather more sophisticated lines than those of the elements of sensory experience. However his mode of operating was similar in that the segments were kept isolated or temporarily brought together strictly under his control. (Residual effects of dissection according to sensory experience and faulty assemblage may have been indicated on the few occasions when he said, 'I don't want to hear' and placed his hands over his eyes or, 'I don't want to see' and placed his hands over his ears).

Early epistemophilic drives

As the early months of therapy proceeded, Piffie showed his conviction that I existed as a maternal object who could be entered and whose contents could be explored and placed under his mastery.

The very literal way he experienced putting himself into my body was shown by the routines he developed for entering the house and making his way to my upstairs consulting room. On entering the house he would make a plunging dive onto the floor. He would then crawl slowly and painfully upstairs pushing his head against each step and saying, 'Come and help me push these plop-plop steps away'. Or frequently he would take out a stair rod and beat each step saying, 'baby, baby', or hold the stick in front of his penis and use it to thrust his way into the room. Just before entering the room he sometimes knelt and spun round as though he were a drill, saying, 'mummy hole' and then twiddled his hand round and round saying, 'wee-wee hole'. Having at last overcome the difficulties of entering the room, he often showed fantasies of finding there the breasts, penises, faeces, urine and babies believed to form the contents of the mother's body.

Piffie also used furniture to construct houses, the rooms of which were closely equated with compartments inside the mother's body, going into such details as to have 'a sneezing room' and a 'coughing room'. The quality of communication in these dramatizations indicated that, at this stage, there was a small degree of differentiation between the house as a symbol for the body and the body itself. Around this time his speech developed quite rapidly, he was also beginning to draw and model. Klein stresses the links between the epistemophilic drives and the infant's striving towards the mother at a stage of maximal oral-sadism:

> It seems that their first object is the interior of the mother's body, which the child first of all regards as an object of oral gratification and then as the scene where coition between its parents takes place and where the father's penis and children are situated. At the same time as it wants to force its way into the mother's body in order to take possession of the contents and to destroy them, it wants to know what is going on and what things look like in there. (Klein, 1932, p. 241)

Extraneous stimuli, experienced as overwhelming intrusions, may be excluded by autistic processes. Possibly for Piffie there was a diminished need to employ these means due to the constancy and the sequestered conditions provided by the analytic situation itself and by finding an object more able to contain the projections of his anxieties. However minor disturbances of the analytic setting caused major upheavals. One such occasion occurred when he saw a window cleaner in the passage of my house, during the eighth month of therapy. Following this he spent many weeks drawing pictures of a man on a ladder, first on the walls and then on paper. He began to count the rungs 'one step, two steps' – then a medley of numbers, improving as time went on. Day after day he stuck these accumulations of pictures to the walls, climbing ladders of furniture to reach ever higher. In the early stages, from time to time, he would break off, run to the window and bang it loudly, shouting, 'Go away, Daddy Man!' Later on he called the pictures his babies as he stuck them to the walls.

The sight of the window cleaner meant to him that his mother-house had been successfully invaded by the penis. This was a state of affairs which could not be tolerated but which could be mastered by great application and by the almost precocious development of his means of control. One might say that he mastered the intruder and took over his skills, including his reparative and creative capacities. But Piffie resisted attempts to assist him to confront this anxiety. His method was to reduce the anxiety to small portions and work it away, rather than to encounter it with feeling and work it through. His advances were in his means of control and by identification with his rival he achieved manic reparation. The experience of rivalry and jealousy was made meaningless and the pictures, which rapidly reached a very high level of achievement for his age, were eventually reduced to stylized indications of ladder rungs and window openings; paternal implements of intrusion and maternal apertures as organized by Piffie.

Reparation

There were many similar examples of reparation by manic means. For example, with the furniture of the room, he constructed a pair of semi-detached houses, one for himself and one for me. He acted that, while I slept at night, he would climb through a magic hole in the wall and enter my house. He then stole my pipes, cutting off my water supplies. Upon discovering this the following morning I was to ring up the plumber in a state of great distress. Whereupon, who should appear at my door but a beaming plumber, Piffie, standing proudly before me with the air of a shining knight to the rescue!

To contrast with this I wish to bring material which I con sider to show a genuine encounter with anxiety, at age five. He wished to copy a picture from a book but failed to do so satisfactorily. He tried to force me to do it for him and when this also failed he screamed, raged and kicked at me, tore up the drawing and upset most of the furniture. He then appeared to collapse and became quite distant. He stood in a corner of the room seeming exhausted and empty, gazing before him with blank eyes, tugging at his hair. Although he recovered a little he remained miserable and distant for a couple of days. On the third day he collected together ten or so pieces of his drawing and care-fully stuck them together again with sellotape. He said, 'Tell me again what happened'. I repeated the interpretations which had been made in the previous days. After each sentence he said, 'And then what?' I reached the point of relating the destruction of the picture to the destruction of myself standing for the mother and his feeling that he then had me only as a broken-up mother inside him. This time he did not say 'and then what?' He said, 'and then I was very sad.'

On this occasion it seems to me that the object was felt to have been fragmented by an attack – not dissected for the purpose of control. The anxiety was worked through to the point of becom-ing understandable rather than worked away to the point of becoming meaningless. The sticking together of the picture was not a manic reparation relying upon the denial of guilt and the stealing of omnipotent qualities. Its genuine nature was shown by its being accompanied by a reintegration of the experience and a restoration of his object, functioning in relation to him in a more valued way than before. Reparations of this nature do not merely restore the status quo but represent 'learning from experi-ence– a step towards maturity which enriches the personality.

Primitive obsessional mechanisms

Much of the material I have described concerning Piffie's phan-tasies, of the mother's inside being like a house to explore and take possession of, may be understood as expressing a release of the epistemophilic drives normal to the developing infant. A great deal of his material however was indicative of the ways in which primitive obsessional mechanisms both powered his drive to possess knowledge and obstructed the development of his comprehension of whole objects.

During the second and subsequent years of therapy, with earnest perseverance, he set about the task of mastering me piece by piece. Retrospectively it would almost appear that he deliberately planned to provide me with sufficient interest and variety to keep me happy and to produce an illusion of change, while privately ensuring that development should be largely arrested.

I will describe two series of activities which are particularly revealing of his obsessional mechanisms. One concerned his tracings and his drawings of the contents of the room. When he was drawing on a paper on the floor on one occasion he made the chance discovery that a shaded area revealed the tracing of a hair which lay under the paper. He was thrilled by this and for many months spent part of most sessions making similar tracings which he called 'carpets'. He was especially concerned to trace over the cracks and nail heads in the floor, using every colour and every combination of colour. He experimented with placing different things under the paper: a piece of string, a rubber, scissors, etc., and every combination and variation and pattern of such collections of items. He also drew pictures of the contents of the room; for example a rubber and a pencil apart, a rubber and a pencil together, two chairs apart, two chairs together, a chair on its side, a chair upside down, a chair on the couch, in the basin, in the waste paper bin, etc., ad infinitum. Such pictures were treasured throughout the subsequent years and were returned to repeatedly. They were touched up, added to, ragged edges trimmed off, assembled to form books, separated again to form other books according to a different method of classification. Later on writing was added to the pictures – but each word of a sentence would be encapsulated within a frame and thus isolated from its context. Such activities have formed a kind of diary and storehouse of memory for him. They also form a museum of the trophies gained from the inside and outside of his maternal objects.

They reveal a concrete form of introjection. He was almost literally taking me over hair by hair, sometimes saying to himself insistently, 'Do it! Do it!' As he rubbed his crayon over the paper-covered crack in the floor he seemed at one and the same time to be rubbing himself into the crack and to be obtaining possession of it by transfixing it to the paper, where it would remain solicitously cared for, but isolated and immortal.

Such activities at first appeared to refer to work upon introjective processes. Later on it was understood that, for Piffie, his activity was a symbolic equation stating that introjection for him was literally a process of incorporation resembling a catalogued collection.

His method of encapsulating me in minute single particles rendered the process almost painless. When, for instance, he took over a hair of my head, I could hardly complain of sadistic violation. Unlike him I was no longer aware of the stray hair as a valued part of myself. It may be queried, however, whether he was unusually lacking in sadism. It is possible that this too had been subjected to the process of being rendered into minute, almost invisible particles. Possibly each picture transfixed not only a particle of myself but also a particle of Piffie's sadism. His aggression, mainly in evidence when being used for possessive purposes, was also employed in maintaining this immobilizing grip upon segments of his object.

A further expression of his obsessional mechanisms concerning encapsulation was shown in a long sustained activity of making parcels. Commencing a few weeks before his first summer holiday he began to spend part of each session placing single or small groups of articles in the midst of concentric circles drawn on a paper. This then formed the wrapping of a parcel tightly tied with string. At first I thought this merely expressed packing up for the holiday but the process continued after the holiday, until eventually a stub of brown crayon was the only item left free for use; a vivid illustration of the impoverishment arising from encapsulation. This activity accompanied a sequence of five holidays. His only explanation was that the parcels were 'too keep the rain out'.

They were indeed water-tight enclosures, designed to ensure not only the exclusion of rivals but also to ensure that no part of me, his object, could escape or have any kind of association or 'intercourse' with any other part of me. The process is the opposite of putting all one's eggs into one basket. Similarly little portions of Piffie were securely deposited in close fitting maternal wrappings.

His activities frequently concerned the assemblage of objects. He made an endless series of cardboard kittens with segmented limbs stuck on by sticky tape. He also painted a series of 'cat shops'; each shop window showed rows of parts of cats; one window showing heads, the next limbs, the next tails, etc., in different colours. These were to be purchased in instalments and then assembled. But having been assembled according to matching colours and entitled 'Father cat', 'Mother cat', etc., the cats would then be divided and reassembled with multicoloured parts and a total loss of identity, which gave him great pleasure. He showed his phantasies that babies do not grow but are assembled from readymade pieces among the contents of the mother's body, his wish to help himself to any pieces which suited him and in particular, his striving to control the composition of his objects.

Frequently he attempted to get me to do things for him. When I would not he often acted that he cut off my hands and fitted them onto his own. The acting became a stylized gesture, suggesting a possible origin for some of the bizarre movements of some autistic children.

When preparing himself for the first attendance at school he particularly strongly felt the need for such action. Day after day he drew the parts he felt he required. My head, his head, my right arm, his right arm and so on. Each time he took possession of my part, giving me his part in exchange and derisively calling me 'Baby, Mrs Hoxter'. Eventually the parts were assembled in two pictures which were Piffie-become-Mrs Hoxter and vice versa. Thus dubiously equipped and clad in my disguise he prepared himself for the severe ordeal of school. In spite of preparing himself for school in this way, he made rapid progress in his lessons as I have already described. Throughout this period there was also much opportunity to work on more normal and neurotic disturbances. Therefore, when, at the age of eight, it was necessary to terminate his therapy for external reasons, it seemed fairly appropriate to do so with a recognition of limited gains and an expectation that further therapy would be desirable in adolescence. There was quite a long period for preparing the closure and Piffie finally seemed determined to face it, saying 'Goodbye forever and forever and forever. I will never ever see you again.'

Discussion of the first period of psychotherapy

It is apparent that Piffie came to therapy at a stage which differed in a number of ways from those of the other children discussed. Prognostically, he not only had the advantage of being the youngest in age on entering therapy, but he was also, from the commencement, the least disabled by autism. Initially he was non-verbal and largely a-symbolic, equating the contents of the playroom with bits and pieces of his own and his mother's body. Yet, from the first weeks, he showed a strong drive to communicate and readily seized upon the opportunity of finding in his therapist an object to contain the projection of his painful and confused states, following which he could experience early processes of differentiation leading to symbol formation and communication. Unlike Timmy his object did not consist of such a scattering of minute segments as to have no discernible structure; occasionally there was evidence of a 'paper-thin' object but the rapid reversibility of inside and outside was maintained as a mischievous game, a conjuring trick of the magician- Piffie, and did not seriously damage his conception of internal space. There remained sufficient boundary between self and object to permit a going in and out of it. Piffie came to therapy with a conception of a lap-like object, ever open to him but nevertheless retaining sufficient rudiments of structure to serve as a container and so to provide a starting point for his further development. Like the other children he had already lost 'maturational mental-life time'. But he could be observed to be making up for this lost time with eagerness and rapidity and this process, during the period of therapy, was not interrupted by periods of mindlessness to any discernible extent.

Piffie's object was indeed segmented but when contrasted, for example, with Timmy, his segments appear to be meaningful portions, with immediate significance in the transference relationship, and with sufficient coherence to enable re-assemblings to take place on purposeful lines.

'Purposeful' seems a key adjective to describe this competent, hard-working and masterful little boy. One rarely, if ever, saw in him the autistic child's passive dismantling of his own mental apparatus. Piffie could collapse in misery and frustration and, when this occurred, the collapse was sufficiently severe to arouse alarm in his teachers as well as his parents, but these occurrences were mainly in response to events which he felt threatened his possession or control of his object. In contrast to the more severely autistic children, much of his ego was intact. Related to this, Piffie's autism differed markedly from that of Timmy and John in that it was an active rather than a passive process, often clearly utilized for defensive purposes. This rendered it much more accessible to interpretation. The processes of segmentation and encapsulation were clung to with stubborn persistence; there was sometimes a mild degree of sadism in their employment and occasionally persecutory and claustrophobic consequences could be observed. Prognostically these features, and particularly the active nature of the residual autistic processes, may have been favourable indications; certainly I found these actively meaningful processes more tolerable in the countertransference, less inducive of feelings of helplessness, than passive dismantling into a mindless state.

To Piffie separateness between himself and his object was intolerable; it carried the threat of death. Any 'growing-up' which implied the threat of separateness had to be forestalled. Development, in the sense of maturation, was largely actively arrested and was replaced by extension of his skills of control, areas of knowledge and dominance.

In early infancy he may have maintained the illusion that there was no separateness by his prolonged sleeping. Later he endeavoured to control his parents and therapist so completely that they might be experienced in a 'parcel-like' way, as a close-fitting maternal wrapping which was moulded around his infantile needs so completely that there was hardly sufficient gap between the desire and its fulfilment for awareness of the deadly gap of separateness to arise. Complete possession of the object, or at least of a segment of the object, was felt to be an urgent necessity to preserve the life of both himself and of the object and it was for this purpose that his obsessional defences were primarily used.

Piffie's early history suggests that the nipple, which he could not grasp to suck, represented an especially dangerous segment of his object. The nipple, which is required as a go-between the baby's mouth and the content of the breast, in itself implies separateness as well as 'togetherness'. Later on, Piffie showed that he felt the nipple, which he called a 'nibble', to be an intruder standing between the mouth and access to the contents of the breast. The nipple-less breast becomes a bowl-like, bowel-like object which he could readily enter to help himself to what he desired. The material will have made it evident that there was little differentiation between the oral and the anal.

His oral sadism was largely projected into the nipple which formed the precursor of later phantasies about the penis. Piffie's attitude was that the breast must be protected from union with this dangerous nipple; it must be plucked out – perhaps like a hair – or wrapped up and kept apart. If the nipple insisted upon its intrusions (like the window cleaner) or if the breast insisted upon its need for the nipple (like the water supply pipes), the problem could be overcome by entering the identity of this intruder and thereby possessing its attributes and becoming the controller and reparative agent of the maternal object. The wish to be the sole supplier of a dependent object motivated many of his drives to acquire skills.

However, the experience of the nipple forms the model for connecting and linking. By denying its existence he maintained the phantasies of entering his object and acquiring its contents. But these contents were then faecal-like segments to be stacked and stored, rather than introjected and integrated. True introjection and integration cannot take place in the absence of the living link.

The failure to achieve introjection and integration of dynamic living objects was a major difficulty in Piffie's therapy. His elaborately developed internal space was organized like a museum of specimens, each scholastically identified, each isolated in its own case, to be kept and remembered forever – but never to be used.

In Piffie's fourth year of therapy there had to be an unusually long break of ten weeks. On his return he acted the part of the prince who awakens the princess from her hundred-year sleep. Charmingly he danced about the room, touching each object and bringing it back to life – following which his sessions could proceed as though nothing had happened. It was not until several months and a further short holiday had passed that he could permit himself to see, hear and take cognizance of the evidence that a baby had indeed arrived in the therapist's home during his absence.

When, at the end of his first period of therapy, he said 'Goodbye forever and forever' this statement was probably not an indication of acceptance of separation from an external object. Retrospectively I view it rather as an indication that he had locked me up in one of his storage spaces. An iron curtain had come down between us externally, and internally he retained an encapsulated object, as lifeless, immortal and as forbidden to access as an Egyptian mummy.

Two years later he returned, this time because his parents were concerned about his manifest depression.

The second period of psychotherapy

On the first occasion he was in tears because the electricians who had been rewiring his home had completed their work and left. Sobbing he told me that 'all lovely things come to an end' and that he could not enjoy anything because of this. He also expressed his acute fears that his mother would die. Subsequently he looked through all his old drawings, remembering them in great detail and was delighted when I also recalled them. There was great idealization of his lost babyhood spent with me.

However, once it was decided that therapy should recommence regularly (although only on a once-weekly basis) he got down to work in his characteristic way. To begin with he was preoccupied with exploring me to master the events which had occurred during his absence. He drew the plans of a block of flats; I occupied one of these. A creeper plant gradually grew and invaded the flats. The boundaries between the flats shifted as the occupants encroached upon one another's territories, exchanged premises, drove out rivals, married, exchanged partners or had children who drove out the parents. In his old style the same picture was drawn, redrawn and altered for months on end. There was also a long series of family trees, showing that I had freak children or murderous children or that Piffie was related to me, but also showing his strivings to control mortality.

For a while it seemed that the once-weekly sessions were sufficient to alleviate his depression mainly by giving him reassurance that I was still alive. At first he mainly used the sessions as a means of facilitating his phantasies of arresting progress in preference to maintaining the ever-varying but never changing omnipotent processes of invasive possession and control. However these processes could now be linked more directly to his equation of separateness from the maternal object with death. His obsessional mechanisms were seen both as a defence against the fear of death and as processes for the primary satisfactions of omnipotent control.

Following long periods of work on these lines it became more possible for him to use his sessions less exclusively for Piffie the omnipotent baby and to be able to analyse more directly the persecutory anxieties experienced at school and the functioning of his psychopathology in his external life. For a long while, however, any threat to the phantasies of omnipotent possession of at least a segment of his object, led to a rapid reinforcement of his obsessional mechanisms.

Anxieties relating to school

Material relating to the severe anxieties he experienced about attending school arose in his first school years and were seen to be continuing, basically unchanged when he resumed therapy. However, it was not until he was about twelve years old that he was really able to talk about school directly in his treatment. The following remarks therefore refer to suffering experienced from at least the age of six, only diminishing somewhat in the most recent years.

He used to put his hands over his ears and run about like a trapped animal at the mere mention of school. He wished to keep his relationship with me as a sheltered area exclusively for the anxieties and indulgences of Piffie, his baby self, and rigidly to exclude all that related to his external life as Christopher, the school boy.

The rigid separation of home and school life was exemplified by his feelings about the school uniform. As a young child he had experienced severe anxieties about wearing new clothes. Wearing school uniform, especially a tie, was a severe ordeal for him. By taking great pains he has avoided ever coming to a session in school clothing. This anxiety has been a further factor in his difficulties about making friends; he used to be unable to bear meeting anyone from school outside school and even later, when wishing to have friends, he suffered acute dilemma as to whether visits should be made in school or home clothing.

He was terrified of other boys, quite unable to join in any kind of game involving physical activity and eminently teasable, becoming excessively agitated if anyone borrowed or hid articles from his desk. A paradox to the rigid separation of home and school life was his insistence that he should be called 'Piffie' at school. A boy had only to call him 'Christopher' and he would be reduced to impotent rage and tears. Piffie the baby had to be left securely at home inside mother; on these terms he could just about step into the uniform and identity of the schoolboy. But there was also a terror of the total loss of identity. It was felt that utterance of the name of the school boy, Christopher, would magically confirm the finality of his being segregated from the identity of Piffie-the-baby-who-lives inside-mother.

He could separate from mother and attend school so long as a part of himself was felt to continue to live within his object, holding both her and himself in a state of eternal union. Emerging from his object, growing apart and growing up carried the terrors of imminent death. Birthdays (before the age of thirteen) were always preceded by weeks of mounting anxiety. Provided that they were kept secret all might be well but anxieties of panic proportions were aroused if anyone, at school or at home, made the least acknowledgement of his birthday.

There was a similar taboo upon any mention of his growing up. If he could envisage himself as an adult at all it was as an orphaned bachelor, existing like a lonely hermit, incarcerated in a shabby room in a state of abject poverty and misery. Later on he dropped remarks like 'When I grow up . . .' or 'When I am at university . . .' and then clapped his hands over his mouth.

During his second period of psychotherapy it was found that Piffie's interests and hobbies nearly all related to his obsessional mechanisms and drives. He had vast collections of useless knowledge. To give only two of many possible examples: from the newspapers he used to copy out particulars concerning the previous day's weather, maximum and minimum temperature, rainfall and so on. He was furious when there was a newspaper strike and his dread of holidays was expressed partly in terms of his anger at the gaps which would be caused in his weather records while he was travelling abroad. He also kept lists of all the items placed in the family washing machine. References to his records could reveal, for example, how many times any particular pair of socks had been through the wash. Family holidays and unscheduled use of the washing machine were furiously resented as playing havoc with his records. Many topics and words were taboo, that is to say the compartments in which they were locked were not to be opened. Thus his name, Christopher, was never to be uttered, but also there were words which must never be uttered in conjunction: 'mother' was permitted, 'smoking' was permitted, but the words 'mother smoking' were excessively dangerous, to be countered by hands over his ears and screaming. In such ways, to a large extent, he continued to be excessively controlling in the home situation although in many respects able to lead the life customary for a boy of his age.

He continued to be fascinated by exploring houses. Both in real life and in his dreams he spent much time investigating the space under the roof of his own home and the adjoining house. He also enjoyed tracing out plumbing systems and talked of secretly opening manholes in the hope of performing detective-like work on the evidence of defaecation or menstruation.

He had an extensive knowledge of geography and particularly enjoyed collecting facts concerning obscure places which no-one else had ever heard about. His envy and rivalry have been almost exclusively expressed in this context. Many of his dreams concerned boundaries and borders, customs and passport controls. He has travelled widely with his family but his long accounts of his holidays used to give no information about his experiences, as they were reduced to lists of facts, such as names of places and time-tables of arrival and departure.

He could enjoy reading books of the encyclopaedia type but had no pleasure in fiction or literature. His school reports indicated that he was poor at comprehension and that his compositions lacked imagination. Comments were made upon his tendency to churn out facts without considering the question. He excelled at chronology and making family trees, researching in the Bible, for instance, to make a family tree from Adam to Jesus Christ. But his school reports indicated patchy performance in religious knowledge and he hated history as taught at school – because it so frequently concerned wars. He was excellent at mathematics.

At first his school regarded him as an exceptionally able pupil; possibly the narrowness of the curriculum leading to the Common Entrance examination and the emphasis placed upon rote memory masked the aridity of Piffie's development. Later on, however, his school reports indicated first an increased awareness of the nature of his educational difficulties and then some improvements in this respect.

Further obsessional mechanisms observed in therapy

When he was eleven years old there was an occasion when I was a quarter of an hour late for one of his sessions. Neither anxiety, anger nor relief were shown in a marked form. He scolded me and soon settled to a meticulous enquiry into the possible reasons for my delay. This took the form of a judicial procedure with himself as the judge, examining, as it were, a list of my pleas for mitigating circumstances. Although conducted with a gentle mockery directed at himself as well as me, this business was nevertheless pursued with serious determination: it lasted for over three of his once-weekly sessions and might well have developed into one of his interminable occupations. He divided a piece of paper into ruled columns and then listed a large number of reasons which might have delayed me. In this way he made a thorough investigation of three areas of my life: firstly my home and family life, that is, delays caused by the possible demands, needs, seductions of my husband, my baby, my son, my daughter, etc.; secondly, my journey to the clinic, each variety of transport which I might have used and the hazards appropriate to each; thirdly, came a survey of my work and relationships within the clinic, the possible demands of a variety of patients and of complications in my involvements with colleagues, of senior, junior and equal status. Each of these eminently realistic excuses was listed, examined, the conclusions drawn that it was no excuse, that I was still guilty. A line was then drawn under the item sealing it off before proceeding to the next conjecture.

This material illustrates his way of dealing with a potential trauma and also the necessity of concentrating upon the structure rather than the content of his material if the interpretations were to be effective. With some reality the appointment arrangements made by me might be regarded as circumscribing an area of my life which he was entitled to use, an area definable in terms of time, space, role and function. At a time of stress, however, Piffie readily experienced the arrangements in a more concrete, less truly symbolical way. His view of the session was then like that of an enclosure, containing a portion of his object, an enclosure which was organized and maintained by the strength of his omnipotent obsessional mechanisms. My lateness threatened to break through the omnipotent control, and once the walls of his enclosure were breached there was the danger that he would be overwhelmed by an invasion of anxiety which he was unprepared to meet. My lateness was therefore apprehended as a potential traumatic experience with which he coped by a rapid mobilization of a yet further proliferation of obsessional defences – boxes within boxes. The anxiety, jealousy and hostility which would have been reactions appropriate for his infantile self in this situation, were never experienced. Each emotional reaction was separated into small particles, rendered innocuous and then put aside, filed away in the legal archives. By this means he himself was spared the experience of anxiety and his object was spared the impact of his anger. For all his eleven-year-old sophistication, his capacity to read and write, to form and examine hypotheses, it can be seen that his reaction to this potential trauma was in its essentials the same as that which he had shown on his first visit to me at the age of three. There was then no reaction of anxiety to the potential trauma of being left by his mother with a stranger. Instead he concerned himself with the ordering and lining up of portions of his object. On that occasion the portions were equated with his building blocks and on the later occasion they were scarcely less literally equated with items in his orderly catalogue.

My lateness, my breach of the therapeutic contract, was also felt to indicate cracks in my own boundaries. With considerable enjoyment he then thrust his way through these to explore areas inside my life from which he was normally excluded. At the same time he felt that my boundaries were demonstrated to be weak and therefore that I was vulnerable to the encroachment of his rivals, each of whom had to be put back in his proper place. His curiosity was heightened by the situation but it could lead to no increase of learning. It was as though he was urged to review the security arrangements of his territory but not to enlarge his understanding. When pursuing the content of the material I found that, for example, interpretations relating to his fear that I had had an accident or to his jealousy of my son, led to no increase of feeling or insight. It was simply as though I had peered over his shoulder, looked into a box and when I had had my say, he would reply, 'Yes – well' and then draw his line, shut up the box, simultaneously shutting up my interpretation – and proceed to the next item. Among all his conjectures there was little room for the possibility that I had of my own free will and judgement chosen to do something else or to be with someone else during part of his session. Although I was judged guilty, really I was guilty only of weakness when others were making inroads upon me. This obviated the need for any anxiety of a true persecutory or depressive nature experienced in direct relation to his object. Neither of us was really to blame, there was merely a flaw in the system and he was fully capable of dealing with this by tightening his controls. Experiences such as this have highlighted the need to focus interpretations upon the processes of segmentation and encapsulation by which the satisfactions of omnipotent control are so successfully maintained. The similarity to the man-on-the-ladder episode is to be noted.

Dream work

When therapy had been resumed for nearly a year Piffie had a dream which concerned *a path made of crazy paving. He wished to take up the stones and to use the ground underneath for a flower-bed. In some places the cement between the stones was already beginning to crumble away, but in other places it was very hard to dig through it.* Piffie's dream work began increasingly to suggest that he was joining me in the task of chipping away at these obdurate boundaries binding the crazy segmentations which crushed the possibilities of fertility and growth. The task often seemed interminable but some dreams of the most recent years indicate increased grounds for hope.

Session at age thirteen

He commenced the session by looking and sniffing into a waste-paper basket and tugging at the handles of some locked drawers, making sure that I was looking. He then produced some crumpled paper from his pocket, seating himself at the small children's table, saying, 'Now for my dreams.' At this period this was the standard pattern for his sessions: first, a preliminary investigation, almost reduced to a gesture, to remind me that such things were still important ; then the production of dreams which he had jotted down to bring to the session and which during the session he copied out in a slightly neater and longer version as he related them; finally, he would end the session by talking about events in his daily life. The plan of procedure was usually perfectly timed to fill the fifty minutes of his session.

On this occasion he had three dreams.

First dream: *He was swimming in an open air pool, but it had no boundaries to contain or limit the water. When he came out he found he was naked and had to go like this to the cloakroom to dress. He was very worried because some of his clothing was missing. He started to walk home but the journey was very confusing. In part he was walking back to his London home and yet he seemed to be making a journey near to his family's country cottage. Luckily he had a compass and could use this to find his way. He now seemed to be adequately dressed again. He passed a garden which was full of cages. Animals used to live in these cages, but now they were all empty, the doors open and the bars rotting to pieces. When he got home there was an enormous queue of people waiting outside his house, 'thousands and thousands and thousands of people '. It seemed that Chi-Chi the panda hear was living in a cage in the back garden. A man was there with a gadget to give an alarm if Chi-Chi attempted to escape.* When Piffie went into the house he found that the parrot (which is in reality a family pet which he detests) *had escaped; it was pecking at something in the kitchen. Its cage which was usually in the back garden was all weak and rotten. Then Chi-Chi's cage seemed to have disappeared. It was very frightening that she must have escaped. The telephone rang, it sounded very real and alarming. On the telephone someone said that Chi-Chi was living somewhere else.* He woke abruptly feeling very frightened.

He found it difficult to account for the vivid sense of fear, first saying with some uncertainty that it was because Chi-Chi might scratch him. But he soon added that he knew that attempts to mate Chi-Chi had failed and that animals kept in captivity were less likely to breed successfully. Following my interpretations he related the second dream.

Second dream: *Together with many boys from school he went to Nepal. They went to the King's palace and rushed all over the place; they ran up and down the stairs so much that they nearly broke them. In the distance he saw some monks who were living in another part of the palace.*

He was very jubilant in telling me about this dream, jumping up and down in his seat with unusual liveliness and giving associations. The most significant of these was that he had read in the newspapers that the King of Nepal had died. He was extremely indignant that this news had not been broadcast. Scathingly, he said that there had been much reported about the recent death of the King of Denmark, everyone knew about that. But if he had not been such a diligent reader of the newspaper he might never have known the 'very important news' from Nepal. When I was interpreting he jumped in to anticipate me by saying, 'and what is more, the King's son is now the King!'

Discussion

These dreams indicate the possibility that the obsessional barriers may be breaking down; this arouses an internal state of both alarm and excitement. The dangers of liberating his objects from the processes of segmentation and confinement are shown to be twofold. On the one hand, if his object is completely liberated from its encapsulating boundaries (like the unenclosed swimming pool) it will have no structure to provide a container, no boundaries to prevent his infantile invasion and he would then be drawn to plunge back into an idealized state of total immersion in his object. However, even in the dream he wishes to emerge from such a state but he fears the loss of parts of himself (clothing) and finds himself in a state of confusion. In the dream he was lost in an environment which was bewildering as different areas had departed from their customary locations. Without boundaries he could not tell whether he was inside or outside of his object. 'Luckily' he found that he had a compass to guide him (optimistically this might represent a combined analytic object capable of maintaining its own unity and its own boundaries). In reality he was at this time commencing to travel about more independently; in association to the dreams he said that he carried a compass with him, and explained that this was useful since, if he asked for directions, people might say turn' left or turn right and he would not know if they were facing the same or the opposite way to himself. In the dream, from the point of finding his compass he regained his clothing and recovered from the hazards of entering an unenclosed object.

On regaining his more mature orientation of being separate from and external to his object, he was then faced with the second group of anxieties, those attendant upon liberating his objects from his obsessional mechanisms. In the dream he saw the rotting cages from which animals had escaped. Those creatures were later represented by the queues of many thousands of people outside his house. This seems to represent the possibility of a return to himself of the multitude of segmented portions of objects, now liberated from their cages of solitary confinement. Before the liberation movement can really get under way a man comes with a warning system drawing attention to the situation. The hated parrot has already escaped from the back garden and is pecking in the kitchen, possibly indicating that the oral attacks are leaving their anal location and 'coming home', to the feeding situation. The main focus of anxiety however concerns the female panda. He is intensely alarmed that he may lose control over this

Chi-Chi aspect of his maternal object. If she should escape from the confines of a frigid and childless state he may lose her to the clutches of a rival.

In discussing the second dream it is relevant that, to Piffie, Nepal was one of the remote and secret portions of the mother-earth, with an exact location known only to a few and accessible only to the highly privileged, in contrast to the contemptible state of Denmark, which was commonplace, easily known to all. In contrast to Barry, for example, Piffie had very sophisticated concepts of maternal structure, expressed in his early years in his body-house constructions, and later on also in his detailed and excellent knowledge of geography. He delighted in collecting the most obscure facts about little-known tiny islands and mountain states, and rejoiced in the superiority this gave him. Also, both in dreams and reality, he was acutely anxious and excited when traversing the boundaries between one state and another, or even one English county and another. His almost compulsive need to master geographical structure points to the effort required to maintain himself and his object outside the Autistic State Proper.

The dreams confirm many previous indications suggesting that the structure and boundaries intrinsic to the maternal object continued to be uncertainly differentiated from the compartmentalization produced by his own obsessional organization. This organization can be seen to serve the purposes of defending himself and his object from the dangers of excessive invasion and also to be utilized to keep a possessive hold upon divorced portions of his object and to exclude rivals. In the second dream it is no longer himself, but the father – King of Nepal – who is responsible for keeping the isolated maternal object safe from being worn out by the incursions of rivals, and, on his death, Piffie can run riot in the palace. This typical oedipal situation, this acknowledgment of his position as a rivalrous son, was rarely manifested by Piffie. It is interesting to note that, at this point, he was able to join other boys in their revels, something which almost never occurred either in dream or in external reality. In the distance however there remained the chaste monks of an enclosed order, the male counterparts of the caged Chi-Chi, who also reflected the aloof position to which Piffie usually retired from boyish pranks. The maintenance of the obsessional organizations often appeared to be a life-consuming activity for Piffie. Internally the King was an exacting ruler, with whom Piffie was usually identified. This slave-driving master constantly kept him to the minutiae of his duties concerning the enclosed portions of self and objects. With regard to these caged objects Piffie customarily behaved as an over-burdened, conscientious but benevolent zoo-keeper, needing constantly to ensure that the cages were secure and the inmates well tended (i.e. not forgotten or lost; forgetting, losing, being late or making trivial mistakes, caused him excessive anxiety). His daily life was run with the precision and planning of a railway timetable: no gaps, no free-time, no letting-up on a long list of daily duties could be tolerated, nothing was left to chance – or spontaneity. This was reflected too in the routine and hard work he put into his weekly sessions, and his horror of running the risk of a period of silence, when the unknown, unplanned for, might break loose from himself or his therapist. It would, indeed, be news of the greatest importance (as he said of the King of Nepal) if this internal ruler were to die and the way to be opened for facing the anxieties attendant upon the liberation of his objects.

The third dream led to associations concerning taking photographs. He said that in a hundred years' time he would be able to show his photographs to his grandchildren, they would find them very interesting. (For about the first time ever he did not clap a hand over his mouth to stifle the slipped admission that he could contemplate a future for himself as an adult and parent, but then his life-span had been manically stretched somewhat.)

Collecting snapshots and studying old family albums had previously been seen to be of great importance to him. He was fascinated that, by a click of the camera, he could immortalize a passing moment. He said his early childhood drawings of the contents of the consulting room were like photographs and was pleased to think that he could always return to them to revive his memories and find things unchanged. We discussed his feeling that the photographs not only literally prevented the object from dying but also prevented it from changing and living. He concluded the session by saying that he was going to the zoo soon, this time he would not take his camera, he really had enough photographs of the zoo animals. With a twinkling smile he added that his snaps included one of Chi-Chi.

Dream at age fourteen

Some months later Piffie gave up sitting at the table for small children and no longer needed to have the remnants of play material handy to recourse to if a silence or gap should threaten the rigidity of his plan for controlling his sessions and his therapist. At this point he was able to use the couch and relate his dreams in the customary manner. In conscious phantasy, however, he had resumed a position resembling that of the chaste monks, and vehemently repudiated the increasing indications of puberty. The following dream occurred at a time when he was struggling with masturbation and fearfully anticipating his first emission.

He dreamed that *he was walking alongside a canal which was cut off from the sea. On the bank there was a shelter made of beautifully carved wood. He supposed it was there to protect people in case the canal should overflow. Suddenly there was a terrible thunderstorm, the sea surged in and flooded right over the canal. It was very dangerous. He fled far away up a mountain side. When he reached a safe height he stopped and looked back, but there was a thick mist; he could see nothing and could not tell what was happening. At last the storm passed and the mist cleared. He returned to the canal, expecting to find the shelter destroyed by the flood, but instead he found, to his great relief, that 'someone had dismantled it'. The wooden sections of the shelter were stacked together and unharmed; they could easily be put together again.* ('Dismantle' was his own word when relating the dream and I had never used the term with him.)

The canal, still water contained within fixed boundaries and cut off from the sea, illustrates his customary circumscribed rigidity, currently exemplified by his insistence that his penis existed only as a urinary tract. The sea and storms frequently occurred in his dreams as images used to represent formless forces (i.e. unnamed, unrecognized) which resisted the confines and controls of his classificatory systems. On this occasion the uprising of his sexual impulses burst through and swept aside the obsessional boundaries. This was felt to be a dangerous threat both to himself and to the maternal shelter whose beauty he appreciates. For a while it seems that he can only take flight. But this time he does not retreat into a further mobilization of obsessionality. He remains intact and in touch with the full emotional impact of the situation and he has a mountain-breast to which to flee; an object which is evidently able to contain his frightened self and to restore his courage to perceive what has 'really' happened. From the safe vantage-point of the mother, the mists of fear clear (and possibly also the threat of an interval of mindlessness?). On recovery he is able to perceive that the stormy waves of orgasm have not caused a devastating state of disintegration. The valued maternal shelter, with its beautifully carved sections, is not so frail as he feared; by utilizing his dismantling processes with love he can protect and preserve it from the stormy inrush of his emotions.

Conclusion

Years ago, when talking about his observation that kittens are born blind, Piffie said, 'Babies are born blind, too. I was blind and deaf until I was three' – the age at which he commenced therapy. He has come a long way since then but my optimism concerning the present indications is tempered by the caution derived from past disappointments. Are the present moves a mere reassembling of himself and his object – a process which can readily be followed by a further dismantling? Or are there indications that preparations are being made for genuine integration? Has there been a real learning, growing experience in this analysis? Or are we both continuing to be engaged in an endless task of shuffling the permutations?

The examination of his apparent development shows the large extent to which he has continued to be condemned to sophisticated versions of the endless stereotypy of the autistic infant. He is able to mobilize his anxieties to extend his techniques of control, he is able to proliferate the items in his collections of pieces of knowledge. But his learning has largely been confined within these limits, static and sterile.

This condition shows signs of modification but is unlikely to change radically until his objects can be freed from their states of suspended animation. But an alive object is an object which can die. An introjected object can survive the death of the external object and can continue to be a source of life. It can foster further growth when, in Bion's terms, the container and the contained are in a state of conjunction permeated by emotion. But an object retained in a concrete system of incorporation is a mere possession, once lost it is gone forever. To Piffie the loss of his object, whether by death or to a rival, is a loss of life. I anticipate that his autism will continue until he can find in his therapist an object who can face the fear of death and so help him to face his own fears. Then his mouth may at last dare to grasp the nipple and to commence a living relationship.

CHAPTER SEVEN

Mutism in infantile autism, schizophrenia, and manic depressive states: the correlation of clinical psychopathology and linguistics[1]

Donald Meltzer

P sychoanalysis in practice depends so much upon the function of speech that we are inclined to take this function a little for granted, until confronted with severe disturbances within it. Such situations make us aware how little this inner mental activity of verbalization, and its outward manifestation, vocalization, have as yet been conceptualized by psychoanalysts for their own clinical use. This chapter is a contribution towards this, meant for use in the consulting room and playroom; it therefore draws upon recent work in linguistics, but cannot claim to offer anything in return to this field. However, it is fitting that the chief sources of conceptual notions should be mentioned at the outset, before turning to the clinical material. The formulation of language function that has been employed rests heavily on the work of the following people: Bertrand Russell's conception of meta-languages at different levels of abstraction; Wittgenstein's view of language as part of the 'natural history' of human beings, and its division into deep and surface language; Susan Langer's view of the musical basis

1   Published in the *International Journal of Psychoanalysis*, 55: 397–404 (1974).

of language which is taken here to apply to Wittgenstein's 'deep' language and to Chomsky's 'deep grammar'; Bion's conception of the employment of projective identification as the primal mode for communicating states of mind, which is taken to be the content of 'deep' language and grammar. It is perhaps well to state clearly that this paper is not framed in sympathy with views which equate the mind and brain, and would therefore not harmonize with ideas which are based on neuropathology, such as Merleau Ponty when he employs Goldstein's observations on aphasia, nor with developmental views put forward by (for instance) Roman Jakobson, which assume that the child learns by beginning with 'one-phonemeone-word-one-sentence utterances'.

But rather than labour further the theoretical debate, it is better to press on to the clinical findings, in order to show how these contain implicitly a theory of language function and development, of verbalization as well as vocalization. The approach may be summarized by considering it as a flanking operation focusing on infantile autism; for instead of describing its clinical phenomenology, clinical material from two schizophrenic and one manic-depressive patients will be set out for the purpose of defining five factors in language function whose disturbance leads in the direction of mutism. It will then be pulled together to show how all five factors are operative in infantile autism, thereby interfering with speech being part of the 'natural history' of these children.

These five factors, which can be seen to operate singly, in tandem or consortium in mental illnesses where a tendency to mutism is present, are as follows:

(a) It is necessary for mental functioning to be sufficiently ordered for the formation of dream thoughts suitable for communication by some means, and not merely requiring evacuation (Bion).

(b) There must be an apparatus for transforming dream thought into language; this apparatus consists of internalized speaking objects from whom and in identification with whom (whether by a process of narcissistic or introjective identification) the musical deep grammar for representing states of mind can be learned.

(c) In the early years, when the lalling impulse is still strong, the child must build up a vocabulary for describing the outside world, so that he may develop a virtuosity in superimposing this surface, lexical, language upon the deeper, musical, language; and so be able to communicate about the outside world.

(d) These internal transformations, inner speech, must find an object in the outside world which has sufficient psychic reality and adequate differentiation from the self, to require the vocalization of this inner process in order for communication to take place.

(e) The desire for communication with other human beings must be sufficient to sustain the continuing process of dream thought formation.

In the clinical material now to be presented, these factors will be variously illustrated: Sylvia, a young manic-depressive, illustrates the loss of desire for communication (e), and a weakening of the process of transformation of dream-thought into language (b); Philippa, an adolescent deluded schizophrenic, reveals a process of forming a delusional object to whom vocalization of inner speech is irrelevant (d); and finally Jonathan, an adolescent catatonic schizophrenic, demonstrates in recovery the way in which the introjection of a speaking object (b) sets going the lalling process (c), once the patient has been gathered sufficiently into a transference relationship to re-start the function of dream-thought formation (a).

Clinical material no. 1

A woman in her mid-thirties, but still looking a frail, pretty pubertal child, had been in hospital for eight years, where she was variously considered to be manic-depressive or catatonic at different times. Sylvia was severely anorexic, and her life on the ward was divided between long periods of lying lifelessly on her bed, and rather shorter spurts of feverish activity as scullery-maid and general dogsbody under the tyrannical control of another patient, Millie, who seemed to rule the ward through a coterie. This Pax Romana, which seemed acceptable to the staff, was only broken when a patient (Sylvia included) would 'go up the wall' and start 'smashing'. The former described primarily screaming assaults on other patients and staff, while the latter term meant breaking windows and crockery. These outbreaks were attributed to intrusion upon Millie's balance of power by visitors from 'the world'. 'If only they would let us alone', Sylvia often chanted, by which she meant also the intrusion by the analysis, to which she was brought by taxi and nurse. She insisted that the system could not tolerate more than two such interferences per week.

As the Easter holiday break in analysis approached, Sylvia began 'smashing' and 'going up the wall', and frequently attempted suicide by various ingenious but relatively ineffectual means when she returned to the hospital after each session.

To the penultimate session she brought two cursory dreams:

(a) *Millie was cutting up lettuce and handing it about*;

(b) *Amy might smash a little tank outside her room.*

Enquiring noises by the analyst or evident incomprehension could draw a few associations from her: sometimes they had lettuce with the meals, over which Millie presided, not cooking but serving. There was no meal in the dream, just lettuce. Amy is a 'smasher', and gets upset at the holidays when the ward empties of less permanent members, or others go home with relatives. The 'tank' in the dream was of glass, big enough to hold about a pint and with gradation marks on the side, like a thermometer.

These two dreams and associations were rather simply interpreted as meaning something like: if only you would let us alone (lettuce alone without other food) and not stir feelings of love (Amy), we would not be impelled to smash up our capacity (graduated, but holding about a pint) for gratitude (tank – thanks – thank you) when left alone at Easter (the empty ward).

I do not wish to plead the validity of this interpretation, but rather to concentrate on its implications regarding the patient's language function. It is characteristic of her, as she totters like an old woman from the consulting room at the end of the session, to mumble either 'M'soy' (I am sorry) or 'Than'y' (thank you), depending on whether or not she has brought material for analysis, particularly dreams. She will weep on her way back to the hospital if she has been unable to co-operate, attempt to throw herself from the taxi, strangle herself with her scarf, or poison herself with secreted pills.

I think one can see clearly the image of despair, like children of the concentration camp, huddled together, submitted totally to their persecutors, scavenging for food and braced against anything that might arouse false hope of rescue. The chant 'Let us alone!' seems to echo and disintegrate into a dysarthric 'lesalon', a mere surly noise as they pull away from tenderness-while the thought becomes reduced to an image, the dream image of Millie and the lettuce alone. Similarly the language of gratitude crumbles into 'Than'y', and the empty baby bottle invites smashing as the reminder of richer promises. One has to understand that for this girl the outside world had become a mad-house in which she had wandered from bed to bed in drunken confusion, searching for an object to fill her with love in the years before hospitalization. It would have needed to be an object without gradations of generosity, that never emptied, that never stood outside the door of her mouth as a reminder of indebtedness.

I wish to stress the way in which the dreams reveal that the propositional structure of thought, 'Let us alone' and 'Thank you', have been preserved in the dream image, but the language function has begun to lose its roots in the propositions and deteriorate into a drunken babbling. But notice that the image has a direct punning relation through homonymity to the crumbling language and stands clearly in a secondary relation to it, a derivative. In the dream we find the relic of language as the archaeologist finds a relic of culture in the debris of the midden. The psychotic world of Millie's Pax Romana has no need of language but only of commands, the equivalent of the whistles and hand signals with which field dogs are trained. Neither the communication of states of mind nor of information about the outside world is necessary, as all ego functions are performed by the tyrant and none by the slaves. But communication is required to ward off the intruders, the analyst in particular, and for this purpose a noise, indicative of the state of mind, will suffice: 'Lesalon! M'soy! Than'y!' One might think that the syntactic structure was preserved, were it not for the dreams which show that it has been replaced by an image with only a homonymous relation to the language. Only the music of the original proposition has been preserved, and this is played off-key and carelessly.

The second clinical example is meant to illuminate a second type of mutism, in which the inner speech is preserved, the desire for communication of information and states of mind is seemingly unimpaired, but a delusional alteration of the object renders the vocalization of language redundant.

Clinical material no. 2

After three years of hospital treatment for depression, Phillipa had awakened from a dream with a full-blown schizophrenic delusional system. It was too elaborate to describe in detail here, but can be summarized as follows: this sixteen-year-old fat girl, intelligent, and rather gifted verbally, had now become the captive of a rich man who had bought her for five pounds from her parents as the subject of a huge research project on schizophrenia. For this purpose she was confined to a movie set where nothing was real, neither the air, the scenery, nor the people; only herself. As everything was being followed by television cameras carefully concealed, Phillipa's every utterance and gesture was studied, theatrical, controlled. However, as it seemed that this control was exerted over her by the rich man and not by herself, she felt no personal responsibility for her behaviour. Her relation to the analyst on the other hand, once treatment was begun, stood in marked contrast to this delusion. It became one of omnipotent control over his words and actions, despite the fact that it soon appeared that she had discovered that the rich man had the same name as the analyst. It seemed necessary for the analyst to restrain his behaviour, especially changes in posture or facial expression, for such irrelevant acts resulted in outbreaks of hilarious triumph over him. With flawless logic she explained: 'You can't seem to control yourself, Dr Meltzer. However, as there are only two of us here, I must be controlling you.'

Although these manic outbreaks initially followed upon extraneous movements of the analyst (such as crossing a leg or scratching an itch), they gradually spread to his analytical activity itself. The effect was intimidating indeed. An inner struggle to overcome an inertia and tendency to remain silent became necessary. But perseverance in the interpretive function seemed gradually to produce a most undesirable effect on the patient, from both the therapeutic and the scientific points of view. As the analyst persisted in talking, the patient tended to lapse into mime; then it could also be seen that she appeared to look at him less and less, until this was reduced to an initial glance at the beginning of the session, after which she directed her attention out of the window. From the behaviour of her eyes, which now commenced a most complicated and bizarre system of blinking and staring that lasted for months, it was possible to construe that she was using her eyes as a camera in the initial moments of the session and as a cinematic projector for the remaining time.

When it was finally interpreted to Phillipa that she was making a photo of the analyst which she then projected outside the analytic setting in order to recover an object of more docile quality, an astonishing confirmation broke the silence of her negativism : 'Pictures are just as good as people'.' Three years of analysis had produced a marked shift in the patient's delusion, though it can hardly be claimed as a therapeutic triumph; from being the only real thing, the actress in the delusional setting, Phillipa had metamorphosed into the director, cameraman and camera all fused together. One might say that she had shifted from a paranoid to a catatonic delusional system; instead of being controlled by the rich Dr Meltzer, she was now in control of the picture of him. In the process of this, her need to vocalize her thoughts dried up, and her conversations could be conducted in mime. Obviously pictures cannot hear, they can only see; but they are nonetheless 'just as good as people'. The point of this material is to clarify the role of the actual vocalization of language. One must not take it for granted. The usual distinction between inner and outer speech does not really cover the possibilities; for one can see that Phillipa's mimed conversations were 'outer', and still silent ; she would have to be described as mute in the analytical situation, not merely silent. Where Sylvia's muteness, or tendency towards it, illustrated the withdrawal from object relations and the loss of desire to communicate, Phillipa's shows a converse process – the achievement of an object, but a delusional one, which had qualities that made vocalization redundant for the purpose of understanding. It must not be thought that such qualities are possessed only by delusional objects; the omnipotent aspect of projective identification probably always has something of this in it. The state of mind, and the image or dream image in which it is embedded, can seem to be implanted intact in the object's mind. To overcome the illusion the child must in some way apprehend the necessity of vocalization and most young children demonstrate only a very partial appreciation of this – with their mothers in particular.

In our third example, however, we are going to move in the other direction, to examine the role of mental content, and how (as Wilfred Bion puts it) it must consist of elements suitable for communication, and not merely for evacuation.

Clinical material no. 3

When Jonathan came to analysis he had already been for five years in a catatonic state of increasing depth into which he had drifted relentlessly during several years of mounting confusion, paranoid anxieties and outbreaks of rage commencing in puberty. By the age of 20 he looked more like a dishevelled child of twelve or a sad little clown, or even a rag doll at times. His verbal responses were almost limited to a tic-like 'dunno, dunno' or 'yeh, yeh', except at moments of rage when he ran about slamming doors and shouting 'Get off my back' or 'Stop fucking me'. Occasionally he angrily insisted, à propos nothing in particular, 'I'm going to have my way' or 'I'm going to do as I please'. His voice was without music, unrhythmic, mechanical. He wet and soiled constantly, masturbated, tore off his clothes, giggled and smirked and was unable to look at people's faces, especially not into the eyes. In some sessions he was completely motionless, sitting with clothes wrongly worn – shoeless or with slippers on the wrong feet, flies open and shirt tail out, hands far up his sleeves. He generally seemed exhausted, although he slept long and deeply at night.

I cannot describe the full content of the first five years of his analysis, but wish here to concentrate on the language aspect. As contact was established, the tic-like 'dunno, dunno' was replaced by occasional runs of words which seemed to refer to dreams and, more rarely, to songs or film titles from the television. Later he attempted to recite the full lyric, so that it was apparent that the content had some meaning in reference to the experience of the psychoanalytical transference. Very occasionally a fragment of memory, utterly dislocated in the time or the geography of his life experience, broke through, but inevitably trailed off into inaudibility and was replaced by 'dunno, dunno, dunno'. As these fragments began to be assembled by the analyst into a history of his internal life, it was noticeable that certain fixed elements, such as his calling himself 'Boris' or insisting that he was eighteen (the age at hospital admission) began to thaw and move towards the truth. The impression was unmistakable that he had begun at times to be able to return from the 'nowhere' of his delusional system, to the time-space-identity world of psychic and external reality; somehow the absolute despair (in the Kierkegaardian sense) of his illness had given way to hope, and separation reactions now began to be very severe.

By the fourth year of the analysis, he was able to relate an occasional dream, a garbled memory, or to describe a recent event at the hospital or at the home of the couple he regularly visited. By the fifth year he was collecting words with abstract meanings, could experience puzzlement about the meaning of other people's behaviour or of his own proliferating compulsions. These involved peculiar modes of locomotion, counting and repetition of words two or four times. But his use of language for the purpose of communication was greatly opposed from within, so that his speech was frequently broken into by his hands being put into his mouth, or picking at his lips, by having to giggle and scratch his bottom, or jump up to go and 'have a wash'. The degree of his enslavement to an internal persecutor could be fairly judged by the distance which his hands were withdrawn up his shirt sleeves.

This lengthy description of a process of partial recovery from a schizophrenic catastrophe, is intended to illustrate a certain thesis about language development and about mutism in the catatonic patient. The illness has involved such a destruction of the internal objects, the basis of identity, that it has carried to destruction with it the capacity to have thoughts and thus the foundations of speech, both in its vocal and its verbal aspects. In Jonathan's slow movement towards recovery of his mental structure and functions, one can discern a slow-motion recapitulation of the development of these two dimensions of the process of speech, albeit with great distortion and pain.

The first dimension, verbalization, is illustrated by the way in which Jonathan was able to introject a speaking, or rather a singing, object, and could repeat with remarkable accuracy the lyrics of a song, at first mechanically but gradually with increasing rhythm and tonal modulation. It was easily recognizable that the content of these songs bore a reference to recent interpretations concerning the evolution of the qualities and relationship of his internal objects and their transference significance, drawn from the analytic inference of his dreams, reports of events and memories, and his behaviour in the sessions.

The second dimension, vocalization, corresponding to the small child's lalling or playing with language, was represented in a rather tormented form in Jonathan's repetition of words and his building or rebuilding of a vocabulary for the expression of his own thoughts and experiences, all of which could be seen to lend substance to a growing sense of identity.

In contrast, then, to Sylvia's sullen withdrawal from verbal intercourse and of Phillipa's displacement of it into a silent mimed conversation with an hallucinated object, Jonathan illustrates a mutism based upon a severe fragmentation of personality structure, with consequent loss of the ability to have his own thoughts with which to think. As the two dimensions of language evolution progressed, he began to have thoughts of his own so that he could feel a desire to understand his experiences, and to ask the analyst to explain their meaning to him. The great difference from the healthy development of a child in its joyousness, is to be found in the quite extraordinary mental pain. For Jonathan, every step forward had to proceed in the teeth of severe opposition from a threatening internal persecutor, as well as in a matrix of resentment of separations and the resulting cruel wish to disappoint his objects.

Discussion

These three pieces of clinical description can be seen, therefore, to illustrate what amounts to a theory of language, its development as well as its pathology, giving substance to the dictum that speech makes 'infinite use of finite means' (Chomsky). We may clarify and recapitulate, by listing the five aspects of mental life which have defined themselves as being sine qua non for language development and continuation. The first of these is the desire to communicate states of mind and information, the collapse of which was seen in Sylvia. The second was the necessity of having an object with psychic reality, and not delusional significance, to whom the language can be directed – demonstrated by Phillipa's switch from talking to the analyst, to her silent conversation with a 'picture' of him which was 'just as good as a person'. The third requirement is the introjection of a speaking object from which, by means of identification, the grammatical music of language propositions can be adopted. The rebuilding of such an object is suggested by Jonathan's experience. The fourth element necessary, is the acquisition of a vocabulary which can be utilized, with a virtuosity born of lalling repetition, for the clothing of dream thoughts in language available for use either internally for thinking, or externally for communication. All these four depend on the fifth element, a sufficient mental apparatus to elaborate dream thoughts suitable for thinking and memory (ex-process), not merely for evacuation (Bion's beta-elements).

This is not the place for a lengthy discussion of how this theory relates to others past or current in psychology, linguistics or philosophy. However, just to locate its references briefly, two quotations may be useful for comparison. Roman Jakobson in *Fundamentals of Language* writes:

> The gradual regression of the sound pattern in aphasics regularly reverses the order of children's phonemic acquisitions. This regression involves an inflation of homonyms' (compare Sylvia) 'and a decrease of vocabulary. If this twofold – phonemic and lexical – disablement progresses further, the last residues of speech are one-phoneme-one-word-one-sentence utterances; the patient relapses into the initial phases of the infant's linguistic development or even to their prelingual stage . . . (Jakobson, 1956, p. 74).

You will see that the theory contained in this paper does not consider that the transition in children takes place via 'one phoneme-one-word-one-sentence utterances' but through the

singing of propositions, through identification and with in
creasing accuracy. Compare the statement by Jakobson with the
following from Ludwig Wittgenstein's *Philosophical Investigations*
(1953):

> Someone who did not understand our language, a foreigner,
> who had fairly often heard someone giving the order 'Bring
> me a slab!' might believe this whole series of sounds was one
> word corresponding perhaps to the word for 'building-stone'
> in his language. If he himself had then given this order per-
> haps he would have pronounced it differently, and we should
> say: he pronounced it so oddly because he takes it for a single
> word. (aphorism no. 20)

This statement corresponds more closely to our theory, and one
is immediately reminded of the many jokes that are based upon
this type of misunderstanding. We are therefore assuming that
the ideas that words are primary artifacts, and that grammar has
an existence as a thing-in-itself, are untenable. Or if I may again
have Wittgenstein make the point for us:

> It is sometimes said that animals do not talk because they
> lack the mental capacity. And this means, 'They do not think
> and this is why they do not talk'. But – they simply do not
> talk. Or to put it better: they do not use language – if we
> except the most primitive forms of language. Commanding,
> questioning, recounting, chatting are as much a part of our
> natural history as walking, eating, drinking, playing. (no. 25)

I will not labour further the methodological errors that
result from confusing mind and brain. Our theory is one which
attempts to deal with language as this very function, of mind
and its natural history. But equipped with this theory, we must
now turn our attention to the problem of the mutism of the
autistic child; and I hope that it will not be disappointing if
this part of the discussion is void of clinical illustration. The
reason for this is twofold: first of all, the relevant clinical material comes from the work of colleagues whose treatments I have
supervised and not from my own observations; and secondly, I
wish to build the concept of the mutism of the autistic child in
a rather different way – taking it on its flank, as I have said. I

do not want to deal with the mutism in the ordinary way as a symptom, deriving its structure, but rather to demonstrate from the structure of the illness that speaking is naturally absent in the autistic child, that it is not a part of his natural history, in this Wittgensteinian sense.

We find that Autism is a type of developmental retardation which overtakes children of high intelligence, gentle disposition and high emotional sensitivity, when confronted in the first year of life with depressive states in the mothering person. The severe impairment of contact by the mother catapults the child into severe depressive anxieties at a time when they are correspondingly deprived of the services of a receptive figure to share this deluge of mental pain and thereby modify its impact. Their response to this withdrawal is a drastic one; but is fundamentally in keeping with a marked obsessional predisposition – that is, a tendency to deal with anxiety by phantasies of omnipotent control of their objects. They employ a special type of splitting process, in which they dismantle their ego into its separate perceptual capabilities of seeing, touching, hearing, smelling, etc., and thereby reduce their object from one of 'common sense' (Bion), to a multiplicity of unisensual events in which animate and inanimate become indistinguishable. The consequence is that, in states of Autism Proper, they themselves are reduced to a type of mindlessness equivalent to organic brain defect.

On the other hand, because these splittings are accomplished along what might be called 'physiological' lines, by allowing a passive disintegration of the ego into natural cleavage by suspension of attention, and not actively splitting by sadistic attacks, the reintegration is very facile, and without depressive pain in itself. When the ego is reunited by an attractive object, so does the perception of objects reintegrate. For this reason, the Autistic State Proper is highly reversible in a momentary way, and does not constitute a disease but is more equivalent to an induced stupor. However, the employment of this mechanism does deprive the child of much developmental experience (in a quantitative sense), and may retard ego development in a very characteristic way. Typically the oscillation between 'common-sense' and 'dismantled' object experience, as well as the factor of relative unavailability of the mother, interferes with the evolution of the concept of internal space, both of self and object, thus impairing both introjective and projective processes. Consequently the ego tends to remain in a very primitive state of fusion with its external object, through the phantasy of clinging or adhesion (Bick). This produces a highly narcissistic form of identification and heightens the intolerance to separation, which becomes an experience of being torn away from its object and its own skin (Bick), or of tearing away a part of the object (Tustin) (Meltzer).

The primitiveness of the ego, the unusual quality of the anxieties, and the oscillation of integrated with autistic states, creates a wildly confusing clinical picture indistinguishable to observation from the bizarre behaviour of deluded psychosis. As they recover or improve, this picture is gradually replaced by one of mixed immaturity and obsessionality.

The mutism has a special place in this context, determined by multiple factors. I will examine these one by one in the order of their developmental significance, relating them to the aspects of language development which have already been defined through the material from psychotic patients.

Mutism is an inevitable accompaniment of the Autistic State Proper, as it is essentially a mindless state in which brain functions rather than mental functions are manifest. This can be misleading where the child has developed some speech outside the Autism Proper, for the language events which then occur within the Autistic State are essentially meaningless, just as they are, for instance, in epileptic equivalent states. This area of the mutism corresponds to the failure to develop dream thought.

The gross immaturity of autistic children, with its special interferences with introjective processes due to the failure to form concepts of internal space, favours failure of language development because processes of identification with speaking objects are stunted. The adhesive type of narcissistic identification seems to encourage identification with bodily rather than with mental functions of the objects, with the dance rather than the song of deep language, one might say.

Later when introjection and projection are more operative, the pregenital oedipal jealousy interferes with the verbal coition of internal objects, rendering them separate and silent. This adds to the tendency to remain non-vocal even when inner speech is developing.

The prolonged immaturity tends to outrun the period of heightened lalling impulse, which seems to dry up around seven years of age. Children who are still mute by this time have a special handicap thereafter in learning to speak.

Because the identification processes are so interfered with and the adhesive mode fails to delineate the particularly human, let alone animate, aspects of the objects but rather their sensual and mechanical qualities, the distinction between animate and inanimate, human and non-human, does not develop or lead to the evolution of internal objects which are a suitable audience for speech.

Finally it can be seen that the poor identifications and the dehumanized aspects of the objects do not encourage the desire to communicate, but only to control or evoke obedience from objects. For this purpose gestures and signals are sufficient.

Summary and discussion

Three pieces of clinical material have now been presented to illustrate five factors which are necessary for speech development and use but are, one or more, found defective in severe mental illness where the tendency to mutism exists. To recapitulate, they are: (a) the capacity to form dream thoughts suitable for transformation into language, impaired in Jonathan and fairly crumbling in Sylvia; (b) the ability to accomplish this transformation, through identification with speaking objects, into the music of deep grammar, disintegrating in Sylvia and slowly being reconstituted in Jonathan; (c) the lalling process of play with words, requisite to the construction of a vocabulary suitable for communication about the external world and to the virtuosity in superimposing this lexical structure of superficial speech on the musical base of deep speech, recovering in Jonathan; (d) apprehension of external objects with qualities of psychic reality which render them suitable as an audience, altered by Phillipa's delusion; and finally (e) a desire to communicate states of mind and information to other people, waning in Sylvia.

In relating these factors to infantile autism, I have described our findings regarding the states of Autism Proper and the impaired personality development in such children outside this realm of self-induced mindlessness. I have outlined the mode of functioning of the central manoeuvre in Autism Proper, the primitive and gentle dismantling of the ego, and traced its consequences, also showing how the disposition which favours such a method of dealing with an environmental failure can lead on to less primitive methods of omnipotent control and thus of obsessionality. This latter, combined with the impaired introjection and preference for an adhesive (Bick) form of narcissistic identification, interferes with the differentiation of the various areas of the geography of phantasy (Meltzer) and thus with the formation of internal objects. This latter difficulty is further complicated in the realm of speaking, by the tendency in later development for the pregenital Oedipus complex to manifest itself as an attack on the verbal coition of the internal parents.

SECTION C

IMPLICATIONS

CHAPTER EIGHT

The relation of autism to obsessional mechanisms in general

Donald Meltzer

The experiences recorded and discussed in this book, deriving as they do from the combination of detailed observation and the panoramic backdrop of years of analytic process, have contributed to our grasp of mental mechanisms in no area so richly as in the field of the obsessional ones. The problem of 'choice of neurosis' with which Freud struggled, by virtue of being formulated at all (one of those wrong questions to which there can be only wrong answers), gave rise to a whole spectrum of speculative theories of one or two factor or even multiple factor type. Stage of development of the libido, fixation points, traumatic factors, mechanisms of defence, mother-baby relationship, sociological factors, heredity of constitution – these and many more have been sorted through in this quest. It might easily be misconstrued that a mechanismspecific theory of autism was being promulgated in this volume, but it would be a mistake which this present chapter should make clear. I intend to show the light thrown on the essential workings of obsessional mechanism by the way in which they are employed in this surely most primitive of all obsessional disorders. Of course, the moment one calls autism an obsessional disorder it sounds like a nosological statement with etiological implications, but it is not so intended. The experience with Piffie has been selected as the locus for this discussion as he presented obsessional mechanisms of a particularly 'pure' sort, as well as in near 'pure culture'.

I must explain what I mean by this distinction from the outset, as I believe we can avoid great confusion by this means. The fundamental mechanism, which we call 'obsessional' after the illness which most floridly illustrates its workings, consists of the separation and omnipotent control over objects, internal or external. This statement seems to require a motivational addendum, 'for the purpose of' or 'to avoid or prevent such and such'. Closer thought, however, will reveal that 'omnipotent control over objects' is in itself a motivational statement, to which one could append statements of secondary motivational development – 'to avoid separation anxiety' or 'for the purpose of preventing the conception of a new baby'. But it is to be distinguished from a statement about the id, which could only properly make reference to source and aim and not to mode and object. The confusion about obsessional mechanisms arises in relation to their secondary deployment as mechanisms of defence against anxiety rather than in their primary usage – 'for their own sake', one might say – as an expression of activity, as opposed to passivity, in object relations. Why then 'omnipotent' if we are merely talking of a form of active relation to objects? Because we can recognize in studying these mechanisms that they operate on the basis of an elliptical phantasy, a breach in the logic of cause and effect which leaps from the wish to its fulfilment without pause to achieve the means of the transformation.

It is the 'purity' of this operation of which I speak in regard Piffie. While, of course, he often employed obsessional mechanisms for defensive purposes, they were gorgeously displayed as his preferred mode for mastering the evolving complexity of his object relations. He was, one might say, a 'born scientist' of the experimental school, an eliminator of variables, an isolator of simple phenomena that could be studied in a sequestered situation. I seem to be implying that experimental science employs omnipotent means, which is correct as contrasted with observational-descriptive science. It is for this reason that the triumphs of the laboratory in the physical sciences fail progressively in the organic ones, approaching near total failure in the human sciences.

The other factor in the 'purity' of Piffie's obsessional mechanisms is to be found in the paucity of sadism in his make-up. He seemed rarely to employ omnipotent control as a sadistic mode of activity, as one sees in severe obsessional illness, paranoia, or – par excellence – in catatonia. The statement of 'pure culture' is, on the other hand, self-explanatory. His transference illness was composed of the defensive use of obsessional mechanisms in massive preference to other devices of defence against anxiety. After all, the obsessional mechanisms, as we see them deployed for defence in the obsessional neurotic, is the most 'reasonable' of all defences against the pain of the Oedipus complex. It simply avoids the pain by obviating the experience of the three-body relationship. The flag of India would be his ideal banner – if the wheel had no rim. With himself as the hub of his obsessional world of object relations, each spoke would be happily isolated from all other spokes – except that they do not seem to be happy, somehow. The phenomena that we are constantly examining in the transference are those thrown up by the unhappiness, deterioration and rebellion, each with its attendant anxieties, of these intransigent objects. Similarly with the manic-depressive operating with part objects, where the separation of nipple-penis from breast seems to be the paradigm of his emotional conflict; the objects deteriorate and become persecutory.

We find that the autistic mechanisms are attempts at a massive simplification of experience, dispersing the experience of objects into sensory and motor modalities, but of course ones which o'erleap themselves and fall on the other side of the dividing line between psychic events and psychic experiences. In fact the experiences seem to be reduced to a level of simplicity that appears hardly mental and accounts for these children appearing to be mentally deficient or suffering from organic brain disease. Piffie had already made an extensive advance beyond his early autism by the time he came to treatment, and what we study in him is the process of personality development, still grossly immature and psychotic, in the structural sense, consequent to the loss of time and ground taken up by his earlier illness. He was certainly the most favourably endowed child of the group from the constitutional point of view, and his progress in the analysis was a steady one indeed, unlike Barry's process of advance and retreat, for instance. But the pace was slowed down by what often appeared to be his capacity for infinite permutation in his phantasy. When he was stencilling the joins of the lino, when he was assembling babies part-by-part – in all these activities he appeared at the time to be capable of eternal preoccupation. One is at a loss to explain the determination of the end-point of each phase – for end-points they happily did have – as one is at a loss to explain the end-point of a manic attack, or of mourning. In these latter cases one may catch a glimpse of the satisfaction of the sadism or operation of the decision to relinquish hope of return of the object, but in Piffie's case each turning-point came unexpectedly, perhaps determined more by something like Mrs Hoxter's breaking-point than by any process essentially internal to the child.

I think it would be useful as a prelude to more detailed theoretical discussion of obsessional mechanisms to recapitulate herewith the notes of a summary of the first two years of Piffie's analysis, which was done in the summer of 1963. I wrote at that time the following:

> My impressions of Piffie are less continuous and less complete than for Timmie, but I will record what has stayed in my mind. This little boy gives me the impression of having been ripe for discarding the paraphernalia of autism, but confronted with.an environment which (naturally) was no longer, as with an infant, equipped to provide him with the kind of simple, repetitive and sequestered experience around which the primal splitting and organization of the personality can take place. My first impression is one of amazement at the concreteness, humour, urgency and florid imagination with which he was able to take the toys and box as feeding breast and the therapist's body as a toilet-lap from the outset, making what is a rather advanced type of split referrable to a somewhat integrated good object.

> While preoccupation with projective identification has been prominent in Piffie's relationship to the room, the stairs and the house, this has not appeared as the central difficulty in the play material. Rather, we have seen that this

overwhelming possessiveness and sensuous demand upon his maternal object have expressed themselves through what I feel is a first derivative, as it were, of the autistic mechanisms – namely, his extreme preoccupation with segmenting (as against 'fragmenting') and reconstituting his object. The emphasis has appeared overwhelmingly oral and has manifest itself in extremely primitive types of obsessional mechanisms of a high order of omnipotence (the packaging, the dining-table drawings, the arranging of the coloured crayons, etc.).

This omnipotence of control appears to be primarily organized in the service of his introjective efforts and we have some reason to believe that it is deployed as a defence against his extreme liability to traumatic experience in relation to the father's penis (the 'man on the ladder' episode). In contrast to Timmie, whose object seemed to be possessed by rival babies the moment it was frustrating or hurtful, Piffie's object seems to be good only when it is emptied of penises, thus becoming passive and easily enslaved (the cushion material, trains, putting drawings in order, etc.). This seems to refer primarily to the feeding situation rather than to the downstairs-with-father toilet-mummy. It is difficult to say as yet what is the traumatic core of the discovery-of-the-penis-in-the-breast type of experience, but my suspicion is that it threatens to explode Piffie's form of idealization of his mouth as the source of all pleasure to the breast, involving or rather subsequent to and dependent upon, a severe denial of biting, spitting, blowing and tongue-stabbing types of aggression.

The manic-reparativeness of this primarily oral organization seems to lie behind much of the 'rubbings' of scissors, lines, nails and other defects in the lino of the playroom. One feels that the scissors-mouth has been split off and projected into the father's penis and that consequent protectiveness towards the breast relative to the penis (again the ladder episode, the leaf-in-the-doorway, the dismantling-of-the-stair-rods etc.) is implemented with crusade-like sanctimony. (Compare, for instance, the Fable of the True Cross, which started as a branch of the Tree of the Knowledge of Good and Evil in the Garden of Eden, was planted in the mouth of the dead Adam by Seth, grew into a tree and was recognized by the Queen of Sheba who predicted the Crucifixion, became the True Cross and was buried until found by St Helen, Constantine's queen, who proved its authenticity by reviving a dead boy by its agency).

In summary, Piffie appears to be a highly intelligent child of whose destructive envy and cruelty we cannot as yet gain any quantitative estimate. His autism seems to have come about rather later than Timmie's, and to have been brought to treatment earlier, after some forward trends had already established themselves, in a milieu not descriptively different in any striking way. In both children the emphasis in the psychopathology appears to be on the failure to develop and utilize the introjective capacities as a means of establishing identity and for coping with separation from external objects. As with Timmie, the dissection of self and objects appears as the primary step in the obsessional devices, but an important difference can be detected, namely that Timmie employs his mechanisms primarily in defence against mental pain, while Piflie seems more bent on controlling the objects of his possessive and sensuous greed to protect them against his splitoff sadism. In both children dependence is severely denied. Another way of stating the difference would be to say that Timmie is bent on evading experience in a way that is so primitive as to fall almost outside the mental realm, while Piffie is determined to control his experiences to obviate catastrophe. Thus he utilises his mastery through thought to deny strongly the difference between internal and external reality. For example, the man-on-the-ladder is clearly dealt with as what-Piffie's-eyes-unexpectedly-made rather than as what-suddenly-appeared-at-Mrs Hoxter's-window.

It is too early to have a conviction that these two children are correctly bracketted in a metapsychological sense, but my impression is that we are seeing the same mental mechanisms operating in relation to different developmental levels of organization.

I am more confident of the answer to this question ten years later. Similarly, time and experience of other conditions in which obsessional mechanisms play an important role have strengthened the conviction that in children whose development is arrested by autism as well as in those who have resumed their development but present us with the post-autistic type of psychosis, a view can be gained of the use of these mechanisms in their most primitive context. The extreme archaism of the personality structure which deploys them, isolated as it appears to be from cultural and family patterns of thought, communication and behaviour, demonstrates in striking simplicity the essence of the operation. This essence may be summarily stated as a device of phenomenological isolation. This term, isolation, expresses the basic principle of the operation, but not its mode of functioning. It has been used in psychiatric descriptive ways in the past to describe the 'isolation of affect' from the content of thought and is truly one of the clinical phenomena of obsessional illnesses. But to describe the mechanism itself I would wish to employ a more transitive term such as 'segmenting' or 'dismantling' (see *Sexual States of Mind*, Chapter 15). It can readily be seen that such terms imply an assumption, namely that primitive perceptual processes involve an integration of the senses at a neurophysiological level, that is at the level of brain, rather than of mind. Much of the laboratory work on perception of Gestalt 'psychology', for instance, is preoccupied with the delineation of these events and their intrinsic patterning. Further, it is my strong suspicion that what Wilfred Bion has formulated, rather than described, as the realm of 'alpha-function', belongs to this category. It is, in a sense, the raw material of mental functioning, the data to which meaning is attributed.

This would appear to be a suitable place for a small philosophical divertissement, to bring together the terms 'mental', 'concept' and 'word' in a manner to make clear that when I use the term 'meaning' I do not intend to imply something obtained by a process of abstraction. I should like to quote a bit from Peter Geach's book *Mental Acts* (Routledge, 1957) and show its link to Bion's idea that concepts are formed by the constant conjunction of preconceptions and realizations, the first thought being an absent object. Geach writes:

> I wish to maintain a far stronger conclusion – that there is no concept at all for which an abstractionist method is adequate. If there were any truth in abstractionism, it would at any rate be adequate for concepts of simple sensible quali-

ties, for concepts like 'red' and 'round'. Now if I possess the concept 'red', then I can perform acts of judgment expressible in sentences containing the word 'red'. This ability, however, certainly cannot be learned by any kind of attention to red patches for any length of time; even if after a course of attending to red patches the ability turned out to be present, we should still be justified in refusing to say that it had been 'learned' that way. We can say this quite as confidently as we can say that the ordinary use of the word 'red' cannot be learned by hearing the word 'red' uttered ceremonially in the presence of a 'red' object – simply on this account, that such a ceremony is not the ordinary use of the word 'red' (p. 34).

Price (*Thinking and Experience*, Hutchinson, 1953) has the rare merit among abstractionists of having pointed out that ceremonious ostensive definition normally plays a rather small part in the learning of language. His own theory is that we learn the sense of words like 'cat' and 'black' by a double process of abstraction; that 'the common feature, e.g. 'cat', in these otherwise unlike utterances, is gradually correlated with a common factor in the observed environmental situations which are other wise unlike. Similarly 'black' gradually sorts itself out from another range of utterances which are otherwise unlike, and is correlated with a visible quality experienced in otherwise unlike situations' (p. 215).

This is much more plausible than the usual stuff about ostensive definition, but I think it is still open to two fatal objections. First, it is integral to the use of a general term that we are not confined to using it in situations including some object to which the term applies; we can use the terms 'black' and 'cat' in situations not including any black object or any cat. How could this part of the use be got by abstraction? And such use is part of the very beginnings of language; the child calls out 'pot' in an 'environmental situation' in which the pot is conspicuous by its absence. Secondly, it is of course not enough, even when language is being used to describe the immediate situation, that we should utter a lot of words corresponding to several features of the situation; but the abstraction that Price appeals to could scarcely account for our doing any more than this. (pp 33–35)

Geach's emphasis on 'acts of judgement expressible in sentences' is a point we have touched on in the chapter on mutism. Here I would emphasize his stress on the part played by the absent object. The point is that the 'mental act' of judgement expressible in sentences containing the word 'red' is not to be confused with the primitive function of reacting-to-the-presence-of-redness which one might establish with regard to bees or sharks. In other words I am taking the position that it is the judgement and only the 'judgement' that is the 'mental act' and that its being 'express-ible in sentences, is the manifestation of its having 'meaning' and being therefore available for communication by means other than projective identification, i.e. in 'symbolic form' (Cassirer), through 'transformation' (Bion).

Now, my thesis regarding autistic mechanisms in particular, and of obsessional mechanisms in general, is that their mode of functioning involves an attack on the capacity to perform 'mental acts' in Geach's sense. While the autistic child accomplishes this by 'dismantling' his 'common sense' (Bion), that is his capacity to experience sensually integrated perceptions to which mean-ing may be attributed, the less primitive forms of obsessional mechanism attack more specific constellations of mental activity rather than seeking a suspension of mental activity in general. The significance, however, of this statement can only be appreci-ated if we recognize that 'meaning' is in its essence emotional. In this conception it can be seen that I am following Susanne K. Langer (*Philosophy in a New Key*, 1942) rather than Bertrand Russell (*An Inquiry into Meaning and Truth*, 1940). In other words, I am asserting that in the autistic mechanisms in particu-lar, as with the obsessional mechanisms in general, the essential mode of activity is aimed at *rendering an incipient experience meaningless hy dismantling it to a state of simplicity below the level of 'common sense' so that it cannot function as a 'symbolic form' to 'contain' (Bion) emotional significance, but can only, in its various parts, find articulations of a random and mechanical sort.* I suspect these latter to approximate, in their more elaborated instances, to Bion's 'bizarre objects' ('Differentiation of the psychotic from the non-psychotic personalities', 1957).

The most flamboyant illustration of this thesis I can cite is to be found in Piffie's manner of dealing with the intrusion of the 'man-on-the-ladder'. The emotional impact on him cannot be doubted. What is so impressive is the systematic way in which he sets about reducing the experience to a meaningless assortment of shapes, perhaps suitable only for apprehension as geometric forms. My contention would be that this reduction was aimed – and without interpretive intervention would have succeeded – at rendering the experience empty of meaning, incapable of symbolic representation and thereby unavailable for internal communication in a manner that could be utilized for memory. It can now be recognized that we are formulating a theory of forgetfulness that embraces a category of mental phenomena quite distinct from those formulated by Freud for the amnesias produced by repression. It may open a window on the vast waste-lands of the past that one encounters in the catatonic patient, empty time-space dotted with disarticulated fragments of recollection and image upon which only isolated words rather than sentences can find a root-hold, as with Jonathan (Chapter 7).

This takes us a certain distance in our understanding of the operation of obsessional mechanisms, but does not yet get at the heart of the mystery regarding their importance in mental life in general. Rather we seem to be implying that insofar as omnipotent control and separation of objects creates a suspended animation and a simplification of experiences into events, emotionality is impaired, and this is the heart of the matter, the reason that these mechanisms are so available for defence against mental pain. But we wish particularly to assert that defensive employment of these mechanisms is secondary, and that their more important and primary function, generally rather hidden from the psychoanalytical method of investigation, is very central to the achievement of a high degree of integration between emotional and intellectual development. While asking that the experience of Piffie be kept in mind, I wish to present two drawings made by a child of nine surrounding a weekend break in analysis. This took place some fifteen years ago and was the first indication I had had of the emotional depth and intellectual potential of a schizoid child who has since developed into an artist and scholar of great promise. At the time that these drawings were made this child was still mute in the analytic situation after two years, sitting at a table with her back to me, drawing away but not allowing me to see.

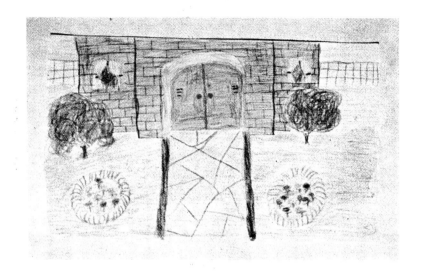

Drawing 1: The house

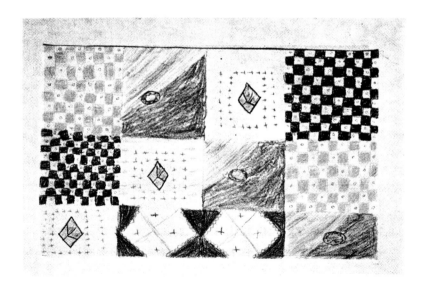

Drawing 2: The dismantled house

Rather as she left each session the drawing was dropped on the floor, much like Abraham's patient who dropped objects from her belt as she walked in the woods. I was thus in a position of carrying on the analysis of her behaviour and of the drawing of the previous· session while she apparently ignored me and got on with her new drawing. At first glance the two drawings appear unrelated, one a stylized house and the other a stylized pattern. But closer examination quickly reveals that the pattern is composed of dismantled pieces of the house drawing.

It is important to note that the two were done three days apart and that I was holding the first out of the patient's view while she did the second. I would also call attention to the fact that the dismantling has been done very carefully – the brickwork, the windows, the crazy-paving, etc. – with one exception, that the flowers in the two beds have been reduced to formlessness of the rainbow colours. I took this drawing, the second, to represent a careful dismantling and controlling of the analytic-mummy in the service of obviating the experience of separation, oedipal jealousy, etc. The only exception to this gentle method seems to be the sadistic attack on the internal babies, the flowers.

That is all very interesting, even rather convincing, but does not in any way account for another striking aspect of the two drawings, namely that the first is rather ordinary and even tedious, while the second is strikingly beautiful and subtle. Note for instance the proportions of Georgian architecture hidden in the pattern. It is also of special interest that the many little naughts, crosses and phi-like symbols did not appear in the original drawing but were introduced the following day while I was interpreting. The child took back the drawing and made these addenda, which I took to represent the way in which the analytic words were experienced as returning life and sexuality to the dismantled object.

As early as 1920 Melanie Klein seems to have been told by her little patients that they were driven often by a thirst for knowledge to explore in phantasy the inside of the mother's body as a world, and the prototype of 'the world'. Search for the truth does not seem to have been a quality of mind which Freud felt to play an important part in the life of his patients and he accordingly underestimated its significance for development. He does speak of the 'sexual researches' of children but an epistemophilic instinct had no role in his conception of the id. What may seem to be a criticism is rather intended to point up the difference of approach implicit in adult and child analysis. While the former works from above, as it were, utilizing the pathological aspects of the personality and their manifestation as transference, child analysis does much more investigating from below, tuning in on a developmental process. This is of course a generalization, and in practice the two overlap in any treatment. Yet it was natural for Freud, faithful as he was to the evidence, struggling against tautological imposition of preconceived ideas, to see operative in adult neurotics the relics of their struggles to minimize mental pain. From that viewpoint every mechanism of defence is a lie. But when seen operative as modulating devices in the development of a child, a very different significance emerges.

Thus it is that we can see, in our researches with these autistic children, that when the struggle against mental pain begins to lose its dominance — and this corresponds generally to the child's turning from narcissistic withdrawal back to a quest for good objects — at that point we can observe the same mechanisms that were used for defence previously now being employed in the service of development. This delicate balance is perhaps best illustrated by Piffie's man-on-the-ladder episode and by my little girl's two drawings, house and pattern. It may also be seen how similar these two clinical episodes are in their structure and how the interpretive process may have tipped the balance in favour of development, gradually with Piffie, almost at once with my far less ill child. It is in fact the gradual aspect, the need to explore every permutation and combination of possible distortion before yielding to the truth, that I wish to emphasize.

Piffie was making slow but systematic use of the treatment situation to explore the qualities of his maternal object in the transference. Of overwhelming importance to him was the suspicion that the daddy-penis was dangerous to the mother and imposed upon her garrisons of invasive, despoiling babies. Only very slowly could he relinquish this idealization of himself as the defender of the faith and recognize his own invasive and destructively controlling impulses and feelings. In order for this sensitive but sensual boy to accept this truth, its dosage had to be minutely calibrated and controlled, and his trust in his object was not such that he could allow it to perform this function for him. I speak here of his internal object primarily, although of course external experiences must have had some influence and certainly his internal situation played a great role in shaping his current external relations, in the transference as elsewhere. Nonetheless, he arrogated to himself this modulating function and this he implemented by his obsessional mechanisms. It had all the earmarks of a laboratory experiment in which many aspects of the situation were held constant in order to study the interaction of the variables. But in a sense Piffie was a bad scientist, caring only for the positive findings and not for the negative ones. He treated the man-on-the-ladder as a negative finding that was equated with a contaminant in the experimental field. The history of science, however, could be written as a constant wrestle with the unexpected. No, at the moment of surprise the scientific-Piffie gave way to the fanatic-Piffie, treating the unexpected as a manifestation of his own supernatural power. The spirit of Jesus yields to that of Paul, and Moses smashes the tablets; the search for truth-waivers and the demand for belief takes its place.

This delicate balance has been described and investigated elsewhere (*Sexual States of Mind*, Chapter 24) with regard to the relation of art and pornography to sexuality in the artist and audience. Where the content of the conflict was stressed in that account, we are now more concerned with the mental process and its mechanics. Tradition has led us to assume that art and science are deeply separated, the former being expressive, a communication essentially, while the latter is an exploration. This has probably never been the case. The great artist and scientist has always been the same person. His explorations of the inner and outer world have always required some mode of publication. His use of inductive and deductive procedures, of descriptive and experimental methods, have always been determined by the opportunities afforded and the materials at hand. These opportunities and materials of course vary from culture to culture, century to century. An advance in geometry may mainly express itself in the paintings of Piero or Uccello. Advance in religious thought erupts as music, metallurgy as sculpture, optics as biology, biology as religious thought, etc.

My point is that obsessional mechanisms, employed in the service of the search for the truth, contribute richly to the equipment of the scientific spirit. But they do, nonetheless, operate on the basis of omnipotence. What I have called the 'elliptical phantasy that leaps from the wish to its fulfilment' does not achieve a delusion, as does hallucination. When it 'gave commands and all smiles ceased', it may have done so out of jealousy but with the intention of creating a controlled situation in which its love, and love-object, might blossom. But it miscalculates in its omnipotence. Its love object does not blossom but withers, the flowers being painted die, the experimental animal ceases, the frozen section dessicates. Experimental science is in this way deeply tragic, and the study of little scientists like Piffie can perhaps help us to see how this tragic element arises from the lack of trust in good objects. This lack of trust is, in the first instance, a disbelief in their capacity to modulate the pain of revelation of the truth to the fragile and vulnerable self. In the second case there is distrust that they would reveal everything, ultimately the 'why', and not merely the 'how' of things.

Descriptive science is more gentle, patient, trusting. I know from experience that psychoanalysis can be an experimental science. I hope it can become a descriptive one.

CHAPTER NINE

Dimensionality as a parameter of mental functioning: its relation to narcissistic organization

Donald Meltzer

It is of interest with regard to the psychoanalytical method that altered views on life-space found expression in the interpretive work long before they came as theoretical realizations. A delineation of the theory has therefore been left very pointedly for the end of this book in order that the clinical experiences upon which it is based, insofar as they relate to autistic children, will have become to some extent part of the reader's equipment. The same cannot be said of the manifestations of simplified dimensionality in non-autistic patients, and this will have to be set right. For this purpose it will be necessary to quote extensively from the pioneer paper of Mrs Esther Bick.

But first perhaps it would be useful to spell out the theoretical formulation briefly. It is our view that, insofar as an organism can be said to have a mental life and not merely to exist in a system of neurophysiological responses to the stimuli coming to it from internal and external sources, it lives in 'the world' and this world may be variously structured. One has perhaps become accustomed to think of 'the world' as four-dimensional and constituting the 'life-space' (K. Levin) of the organism. From the psychoanalytical viewpoint this life-space may be said to comprise the various compartments of the 'geography of phantasy' (Meltzer) moving on the dimension of time. This geography is ordinarily organized into four compartments: inside the self; outside the self; inside internal objects; inside external objects; and to these may sometimes, perhaps always, be added the fifth compartment, the 'nowhere' of the delusional system, outside the gravitational pull of good objects. The dimension of time on the other hand can be recognized to have a development from circularity to oscillation and finally to the linear time of 'life-time' for the individual, from conception to death.

We have now become aware that the spatial dimensionality also has a development, a view probably in fundamental accord with the ideas of Bion as described mainly in *Transformations* (1967). The viewpoint we wish to adopt here is perhaps more immediately clinical and purely psychoanalytical than Bion's, for he is more concerned with thinking and thinking-about-thinking, while we are absorbed mainly with the sources of emotionality in perception and experience. But that the two vertices are complementary seems fairly certain.

This developmental view of dimensionality in the view-of-the-world (which we would not wish to confuse with Weltanschauung, a far more abstract and philosophic idea) does probably take us back to processes of differentiation and organization proximal to the splitting-and-idealization of self and object. Melanie Klein viewed this as the first definitive step in healthy development, a view with which Roger MoneyKyrle, describing the inner logical necessity of development, is in accord. It would seem to us that splitting-and-idealization would arise as a logical necessity somewhere between the establishment of two-dimensionality and before the transition to three-dimensionality. Let us see if we can justify this view by describing the organization of experience at these various levels. It will be clearer if we follow the chronology of development rather than the order in which the realizations arose in our clinical work.

One-dimensionality

Freud's original systematic theory as expressed in the *Project*, the seventh chapter of the *Traumdeutung* or the *Three Essays* is essentially a description of one-dimensionality: source, aim and object of neurophysiologically and genetically determined drive patterns. A linear relationship of time–distance between self and object would give rise to a 'world' which had a fixed centre in the self and a system of radiating lines having direction and distance to objects which were conceived as potentially attractive or repellent. It would only seem fortuitous, in such a world, if moving away from one object simultaneously moved the self towards another. Time would be indistinguishable from distance, a compound of distance and velocity, one might say, closure-time. It is not a world conducive to emotionality except of the simplest polarized sort. Gratification and fusion with the object would be undifferentiated. We have suggested in this book a picture of Autism Proper which is consonant with the reduction of experience to a one-dimensional world, which we have characterized as substantially mindless, consisting of a series of events not available for memory or thought.

Two-dimensionality

When the significance of objects is experienced as inseparable from the sensual qualities that can be apprehended of their surfaces, a conception of the self must necessarily be limited. The self will be experienced also as a sensitive surface, a view not significantly different from Freud's view of the ego as put forward in 'The ego and the id'. This sensitive surface may be marvellously intelligent in the perception and appreciation of the surface qualities of objects, but its aims will necessarily be curtailed by an impoverished imagination, as it will have no means for constructing in thought objects or events different from those it has actually experienced. In the language of Bion, it would have no means for distinguishing between an absent good-object and the presence of a persecuting absent-object. The reason for this limitation of thought and imagination would reside in the lack of an internal space within the mind in which phantasy as trial action, and therefore experimental thought, could take place.

Furthermore the self which was living in a two-dimensional world would be impaired both in memory and desire, or foresight, for the same reason. Its experiences could not result in the introjection of objects or introjective modification of its existing objects. It could not therefore conduct in thought experiments in regression or progression from which the memory of past events could be reconstructed more or less accurately, and future possibilities adumbrated with some degree of conviction. Its relationship to time would be essentially circular, since it would be unable to conceive of enduring change, and therefore of development – or cessation. Circumstances which threaten this changelessness would tend to be experienced as break-down of the surfaces – cracking, tearing, suppuration, dissolution, lichenification or ichthyotic desensitizing, freezing numbness, or a diffuse, meaningless, and therefore tormenting sensation such as itching.

Three-dimensionality

Once the object has been experienced as resisting penetration, so that the emotional problems no longer seem merely ones of being on one side or the other of a paper-thin object (front-side and back-side for instance), the stage is set, as we have seen in the development of John and Barry in particular, for the conception to arise of orifices in object and self. The struggle can then commence concerning the guarding or closing of these orifices, which are conceived as natural rather than forced or torn. With the inception of this new struggle the entire view-of-the-world rises to a new level of complexity, the three-dimensional one, of objects, and, by identification, the self, as containing potential spaces.

The potentiality of a space, and thus the potentiality of a container, can only be realized once a sphincter-function has become effective. It is with the evolution and development of these sphincters that so much of Barry's analysis was concerned. His material shows with particular clarity that the capacity of the object to protect and thus to control its own orifices is a precondition for the self to make a move in that direction, of continence as well as of resistance to aggressive penetration. But insofar as the inside of an object also persists in having the meaning of a prior state of mind, for the feeling of being adequately contained is a precondition for the experience of being a continent container, the movements in phantasy of getting into and out of an object necessarily have a significance with regard to the conception of time. Time which had been indistinguishable from distance in the one-dimensional mindlessness and had achieved a certain vague continuity or circularity from moving from point to point on the surface of a two-dimensional world, now begins to take on a directional tendency of its own, a relentless movement from inside to outside the object. But the continued operation of omnipotence fashions the phantasy of projective identification. By this means not only is there asserted the reversibility of differentiation of self from object but also, as a corollary, a claim is put forward concerning the reversibility of the direction of time. Oscillatory time thus arises in the mind's conceptions of 'the world' and must wait upon the painful, and never fully completed, movement of relinquishment of projective identification in order to become one-directional. Time then becomes the implacable spouse of Fate, that imponderable random factor in the outside world.

Four-dimensionality

It is only once the struggle against narcissism has been mounted and the omnipotence with which intrusion and control is imposed upon good objects in the inner and outer worlds has diminished, that the realization of a four-dimensional world can commence. This is of course of the most crucial importance, as we have seen with Barry and Piffie, for it carries in its wake the vision of development as a possibility. Where envy could find no assuagement and jealousy no balm but in the assertion of the will, now a new hope can arise. And this new hope inspires the process of a new type of identification, which Freud discovered and described in 'The ego and the id'. But introjective identification is a very different affair from the narcissistic ones. Relinquishment is its precondition, time is its friend and hope is its hallmark.

Narcissistic identification

The concept of identification rather tiptoes into Freud's thought; starting perhaps with Dora, more noticeable in the original notes of the Rat-man, it begins to assume the shape of a concept in the discussion of Leonardo, Schreber, and the Wolf-man. But only in *Mourning and Melancholia* is it given full status. By this time the recognition of narcissism was well established and Freud was gradually taking stock of narcissistic phenomena, among which he was able to recognize that a type of identification quite different from that which arose as the 'heir' to the Oedipus complex, marked the early period. He was inclined to think that this primitive form of identification functioned prior to object choice or was in a sense identical with it. The mental mechanics of identification processes, however, remained undescribed despite Ferenczi's delineation of introjection until Melanie Klein's 1946 paper on schizoid mechanisms, among which she listed for the first time the phantasy underlying projective identification.

To a preponderant degree the work of her followers in the next thirty years consisted of investigating the phenomenology of projective identification. This range of phenomena which came into view with the help of the new conceptual tool had a great impact on technique insofar as it gave substance to the idea of the psychotic transference and brought its modification by interpretation within range. It was generally assumed by those working along these lines that projective identification was the mechanism of narcissistic identification and could be confidently looked to as the basis of hypochondria, confusional states, claustrophobia, paranoia, psychotic depression and perhaps some psycho-somatic disorders. In this way the history of projective identification is rather similar to that of repression, having gradually to yield its exclusive position as other mechanisms of defence were discovered. In describing the second mechanism of narcissistic identification, adhesive identification, Esther Bick has opened the way. In this chapter we wish to explore the concept in its relation to two-dimensionality, suggesting that it stands in a specific relation to this view-of the-world, while projective identification is the mechanism par excellence of narcissistic identification in a three-dimensional world. Introjective identification would then be seen as coming into play to raise the mental life out of the sphere of narcissism in specific connection with four-dimensionality.

The phenomenology of adhesive identification in autism

The children that we have studied present a kaleidoscope of clinical phenomena which it has been our task to sort out.

These have been grouped in the clinical descriptions generally under the headings of *Autism Proper, Post-autistic Obsessional Psychosis*, and *Post-autistic Immaturity*. Timmy's material illustrated the first category, John and Barry the second, and Piffie the third. The struggle to attain three-dimensionality was suggested in Timmy's case but most clearly brought out in the treatment process with Barry. This child's slow and arduous progress showed most clearly the parallel movement in the development of the object in respect of the skin-container function and the development of the self with regard to the essentials of humanity. It is therefore with Barry's material that we wish to concern ourselves in describing the phenomenology of adhesive identification that can be seen in retrospect to have characterized his evolution.

Dependence. Unlike projective identification which tends to give rise to a delusion of independence due to loss of the differentiation between adult and infantile capabilities, adhesive identification seems to produce a type of clinging dependence in which the separate existence of the object is unrecognized. Tyrannical control seems not quite a correct description as the need for coercion is barely conceived. Rather the services of the parental figures are absolutely taken for granted in much the same way that one ordinarily takes for granted the obedience of one's hand to one's intentions. This of course plays a part in the impaired impulse to communicate, as described in Chapter 7. The autistic child will naturally take an adult's hand to impel it to perform a service.

Separation – collapse. While the child in projective identification will experience the refusal of his tyranny as a threat to his omnipotence and reduplicate his efforts, a similar refusal in the case of adhesive identification produces collapse, as if torn off and thrown away by the object. This can be seen very clearly in John at the holidays and particularly in Barry at the first summer holiday which he spent bandaging himself – and his object.

Thus for the adhesively identified child refusal of control by an external object and its disappearance are virtually indistinguishable, while for the child in projective identification the

experience of separation can be completely obviated by turning to intrude into his internal object in the absence of the
external one. Thus the comparison between the two seems fairly
paradoxical, for the adhesively identified child, by virtue of the
relatively soft and clinging mimicry, does not appear to be so
tyrannical, nor, consequently, so obviously needy. The acuteness
of the collapse is all the more surprising if notice of impending
separation has not been given to which the child could react
with anxiety. It was of the utmost importance in the treatment
of the children in this group that they should not be allowed to
ignore the approach of a holiday break. Most of the therapists
adopted both visual and verbal means for ensuring the impact
of this information.

Empty-headedness. One of the most characteristic manifestations of projective identification, namely the delusion of
knowledge or of clarity of insight, appears to be absent in the
case of adhesive identification. In fact the contrary seems to be
the case, that just as this delusional sense of knowledge often
misleads one to overestimate the intelligence of the pseudo-
mature child, so one can easily underestimate that of the adhesively identified one. Their identification processes seem to lead
so much more in the direction of mimicry of the surface appearance and behaviour of their objects than of their mental states
or attributes that they often appear to be rather empy-headed,
as one may see in athletes and dancers, actors and models.

Caricaturing. One of the characterological features of people
who greatly employ projective identification is the degree to
which they present to the world a hostile caricature of their
objects. The demeanour of the tranvestite is an extreme example
of this but it can be seen in any case of pseudo-maturity. On
the contrary the mimicry of the adhesively identified presents
a caricature, but one that is far from hostile. Rather it has the
quality of a diminutization, with all the charm that this tends
to imply. The way in which John began automatically to tap
in rhythm with the leaf sweeper, or to sway with the tree, are
examples. When this sort of child is seen walking holding an
adult's hand the blending together takes on a most appealing
pas-de-deux quality.

But when we move into the realm of intelligent behaviour, the picture loses its charm. Here again the projectively identified child may slightly annoy with the pretentiousness or pomposity of his vocabulary or demeanour, or amuse us by its coarseness, depending on the quality of his object. But the adhesively identified child tends to startle us with the unintelligent echoing of his internal or external object. This was seen frequently with Timmie and John, where alterations in tone of voice as well as the absence of the first person pronoun indicated the parroting.

Other phenomena characteristic of adhesive identification could be cited at length, but as it is not our purposes here to expound but only to make explicit the concept, we must now turn our inquiry in another direction. This takes us into the area of compensatory efforts seen in the ego-functions where two-dimensionality is still very prevalent. In order to do this, I will quote extensively from Mrs Bick's 1968 paper, 'The experience of the skin in early object relations':

> The thesis is that in its most primitive form the parts of the personality are felt to have no binding force amongst themselves and must therefore be held together in a way that is experienced by them passively, by the skin functioning as a boundary. But this internal function of containing the parts of the self is dependent initially on the introjection of an external object, experienced as capable of fulfilling this function. Later, identification with this function of the object supersedes the unintegrated state and gives rise to the fantasy of internal and external spaces. Only then is the stage set for the operation of primal splitting and idealization of self and object as described by Melanie Klein. Until the containing functions have been introjected, the concept of a space within the self cannot arise. Introjection, i.e. construction of an object in an internal space is therefore impaired. In its absence, the function of projective identification will necessarily continue unabated and all the confusions of identity attending it will be manifest.
>
> The stage of primal splitting and idealization of self and object can now be seen to rest on this earlier process of containment of self and object by their respective 'skins'.

The fluctuations in this primal state will be illustrated in case material from infant observation, in order to show the difference between unintegration as a passive experience of total helplessness, and disintegration through splitting processes as an active defensive operation in the service of development. We are, therefore, from the economic point of view, dealing with situations conducive to catastrophic anxieties in the unintegrated state as compared with the more limited and specific persecutory and depressive ones.

The need for a containing object would seem, in the infantile unintegrated state, to produce a frantic search for an object – a light, a voice, a smell, or other sensual object – which can hold the attention and thereby be experienced, momentarily at least, as holding the parts of the personality together. The optimal object is the nipple in the mouth, together with the holding and talking and familiar smelling mother.

Material will show how this containing object is experienced concretely as a skin. Faulty development of this primal skin function can be seen to result either from defects in the adequacy of the actual object or from fantasy attacks on it, which impair introjection. Disturbance in the primal skin function can lead to a development of a 'second-skin' formation through which dependence on the object is replaced by a pseudo-independence, by the inappropriate use of certain mental functions – or perhaps innate talents – for the purpose of creating a substitute for this skin container function. The material to follow will give some examples of 'second-skin' formation.

Infant observation: Baby Alice

One year of observation of an immature young mother and her first baby showed a gradual improvement in the 'skin-container' function up to twelve weeks. As the mother's tolerance to closeness to the baby increased, so did her need to excite the baby to manifestations of vitality lessen. A consequent diminution of unintegrated states in the baby could be observed. These had been characterized by trembling, sneezing, and disorganized movements. There followed a move to a new house in a still unfinished condition. This disturbed severely the mother's holding capacity and led her to a withdrawal from the baby. She began feeding whilst watching television, or at night in the dark without holding the baby. This brought a flood of somatic disturbance and an increase of unintegrated states in the baby. Father's illness at that time made matters worse and the mother had to plan to return to work. She began to press the baby into a pseudo-independence, forcing her onto a training-cup, introducing a bouncer during the day, whilst harshly refusing to respond to the crying at night. The mother now returned to an earlier tendency to stimulate the child to aggressive displays which she provoked and admired. The result by six and a half months was a hyperactive and aggressive little girl, whom her mother called 'a boxer' form her habit of pummelling people's faces. We see here the formation of a muscular type of self-containment 'second-skin' in place of a proper skin container.

Analysis of a schizophrenic girl: Mary

Some years of analysis, since age three-and-a-half, have enabled us to reconstruct the mental states reflected in the history of Mary's infantile disturbance. The facts are as follows: a difficult birth, early clenching of the nipple but lazy feeding, bottle supplement in the third week but on the breast until eleven months, infantile eczema at four months with scratching until bleeding, extreme clinging to mother, severe intolerance to waiting for feeds, delayed and atypical development in all areas.

In the analysis, severe intolerance to separation was reflected from the start, as in the jaw-clenched systematic tearing and breaking of all materials after the first holiday break. Utter dependence on the immediate contact could be seen and studied in the unintegrated states of posture and motility on the one hand, and thought and communication on the other, which existed at the beginning of each session, improving during its course, to reappear on leaving. She came in hunched, stiff-jointed, grotesque like a 'sack of potatoes' as she later called herself, and emitting an explosive 'SSBICK' for 'Good morning, Mrs Bick'. This 'sack of potatoes' seemed in constant danger of spilling out its contents, partly due to the continual picking of holes in her skin representing the 'sack' skin of the object in which parts of herself – the 'potatoes' were contained (projective identification). Improvement from the hunched posture to an erect one was achieved, along with a lessening of her general total dependence, more through a formation of a second skin based on her own muscularity than through identification with a containing object.

Analysis of an adult neurotic patient

The alternation of two types of experience of self – the 'sack of apples' and the 'hippopotamus' – could be studied in regard to quality of contact in the transference and experience of separation, both being related to a disturbed feeding period. In the 'sack of apples' state, the patient was touchy, vain, in need of constant attention and praise, easily bruised and constantly expecting catastrophe – such as a collapse when getting up from the couch. In the 'hippopotamus' state of [another, adult] patient, he was aggressive, tyrannical, scathing, and relentless in following his own way. Both states relate to the 'second-skin' type of organization, dominated by projective identification. The 'hippopotamus' skin, like the 'sack', reflects the object's skin inside which he existed, whilst the thin-skinned, easily bruised, apples inside the sack represented that state of parts of the self which were inside this insensitive object.

Analysis of a child: Jill

Early in the analysis of a five-year-old child, whose feeding period had been characterized by anorexia, skin-container problems presented themselves, as in her constant demand of mother during the first analytic holiday that her clothes be firmly fastened, her shoes tightly laced. Later material showed her intense anxiety and need to distinguish herself from toys and dolls, about which she said: 'Toys are not like me, they break to pieces and don't get well. They don't have a skin. We have a skin!'

This is the substance of the paper which opened up the problem of un-integration as contrasted with dis-integration, relating it to defective containment. Mrs Bick has traced some of the compensatory efforts of pathological self-containment. In describing post-autistic psychosis (Barry, for instance) we have also outlined a state of un-integration, while Autism Proper has been viewed as an extremely primitive form of dis-integration.

*The phenomenology of adhesive identification in neurotic
and psychotic patients*

I have quoted at such length from Mrs Bick's paper because it not only delineates the problem of the skin-container function and its relation to ego strength but also goes some distance in scouting out the methods by which this ego strength can be simulated in what she calls 'second-skin' function. I have earlier described some of the findings with the children of this study which illustrate the various aspects of impaired mental function which we think are contingent upon the failure to achieve three-dimensionality in the conception of self and object which is the necessary pre-condition to the container-function. Where Mrs Bick has demonstrated a step in mental organization of experience proximal in time to the operation of splitting-and idealization (which in its turn is preconditional to splitting-and-projective-identification), we are attempting a further step. Instead of defects in the container-function of the object we are attempting to describe defects in the conception-of-the-object-as-a-container, namely the two-dimensional conception. Clinical experience of neurotic and psychotic patients enables us to amplify these descriptions by another phenomenon which is linked on the one hand to preoccupation with surface phenomena between self and objects and on the other hand to the impairment of time sense resulting from a failure to conceive of enduring change, circular time. I will describe this in a way that is intended to stand between mindlessness and depth in the experience of life, namely shallowness.

Shallowness as a character organization

Clinical material

A handsome and well-built young woman who came to analysis some years after the death of one of her parents demonstrated in her demeanour a social breeziness, skill in chatty repartee and scattering of interests which stood in marked contrast on the one hand to the qualities of her childhood environment and on the other to her aspirations. She greatly admired people of passionate conviction, devotion, faithfulness and a sense of urgency, and was quite aware of her utter lack of these qualities. Her relation to time was vague, though not unpunctual. Rather she noted some sort of painless 'waiting' which her friends also noticed and teased her about, that she was always to be found sitting behind her newspaper. Others had to seek her out, which they did, for she was engaging and friendly, but she did not arouse strong feelings in others except by her sexual attractiveness. Her most intense emotional response was elicited by questions of 'good taste' in matters of dress, house furnishing and social deportment. What she noticed and was impressed by in others was in the first instance good looks and dress, so that it was apparent that her relation to her skin was very little distinguished from that to her clothing.

During the second year of the analysis she developed several mild skin disorders, and it was noticeable that her relation to the analyst and to her general practitioner were alike indistinguishable from that to her hairdresser if he had done a bad job. She clearly felt more dirtied than diseased, more humiliated than worried, irritable and impatient rather than concerned with the treatment of the skin disorder. It soon became apparent in the analysis that a narcissistic organization of enslavement to a big-sister-in-law aspect of herself was the determining factor in the perseverance of this attitude. But while it served to elucidate its form vis à vis the outside world, it did not really account for its fundamental quality, the shallowness.

Some years of analysis brought many gains in the organization of her personality in other respects. She married, had children, felt happy – but not content, for she noticed that her interests were still wide and shallow, her activities contingent upon the demands of others rather than inner-directed, and no feeling of individual strength and identity seemed to accrue. The breaking through of this shallowness came somewhat suddenly at times, only to disappear with equal promptness. A flood of love in the transference would take her back for a moment to equally rare moments in her childhood relation to her mother, then disappear and be replaced by recollections of getting her dress dirty or wetting herself. An interesting dream illustrates this process rather eloquently. In the dream *she and her little girl seemed to be living at the house of her daily woman and she felt both greatly impressed by the quality of the life in the household and the immense amount of work that Mrs C managed to do. And the front garden was rather beautiful (like that at the analyst's consulting room) and her little girl was sliding on the surface of the ice in a littlefish-pond. But suddenly she fell through the ice and the patient, in a moment of intense pain rather than panic, threw herself into the water to rescue her. Somehow when she emerged only the front of her dress was a bit wet, as if she had wetted herself as when a child.*

The process of contact with more intense feelings progressed hand in hand with another aspect of the analytic work, namely the investigation of her envious voyeurism. It was necessary over and over to show her the evidence that her minute scrutiny of the surface qualities of the analyst's life – his clothes, the consulting room, house, garden, etc. – were in fact accompanied by damaging intrusions, as illustrated in the dream of the child falling through the surface of the ice, impairing her object and reducing it to the 'daily woman' type of servant who came to clean her house, was paid and dismissed from thought. Only very gradually did the omnipotence of this voyeurism diminish and the appreciation of the fundamental privacy and mysteriousness of her objects arise.

This case material may help to demonstrate how a particular area of the infantile unconscious relationship to the internal mother as whole object (Mrs C the daily-woman) and part-object breast (fish pond) can be impaired in regard to skincontainer and dimensionality undermining the strength and vitality of the personality as an entirety while hardly producing any effects that could be identified from the purely psychiatric descriptive point of view. The patient in question stands in a startling contrast to Barry, say, and to bring them together serves to illustrate the importance of economic factors and of the total matrix of personality within which a particular area of defect is found to be embedded. In the case described the twodimensionality was not a primary developmental failure but had been invoked as a defensive organization regressively in childhood in the face of the genital Oedipus complex and reinforced in late adolescence upon the sudden death of a parent. The question must now be raised, in what way does the two-dimensionality that we are describing differ from the denial of psychic reality, seen in latency for instance, with its common-sensicalness, lack of imagination and impoverishment of affect.

Two-dimensionality versus denial of psychic reality

Great confusion exists in the psychoanalytical literature between the description of impaired mental functions and the impaired consciousness of mental events. Freud's attempts to remedy this by the differentiation of 'denial' from 'negation' and of 'suppression' from 'repression' (1910 and 1925) went some distance to set things right, but the confusion tends to proliferate. The denial of psychic reality, as a concept, tends to straddle these two categories in an unfortunate way, for by it we tend to mean both that the refusal of interest and attention to events of the inner world impairs the consciousness of them but also that this lack of attention facilitates certain operations of omnipotence.

By speaking of two-dimensionality on the other hand we appear to be making no statement referrable to consciousness, interest or attention at all, but purely with regard to the organization of perceptual processes concerning self and objects, the 'world'. By 'shallowness', for instance, I do not mean to refer in particular to the thinness of the emotionality but rather to imply that this same thinness is a necessary consequence of the surface to surface relation to objects.

Another point of importance concerns the question of ego strength. It seems more than likely that in describing the container–contained function (Bion) and the 'skin-container' function (Bick), these two authors have made a deep sally into the important and mysterious problem of ego-strength. While Freud could find the answer to the question of how people keep from falling ill by discovering the role of splitting processes, Bion and Bick have probably gone some considerable way toward discovering how people develop real strength.

CHAPTER TEN

Conclusion

Donald Meltzer

By the time that a book has written itself and its various parts been put together, perhaps in particular, as in the present instance, when several people have worked together and separately on it, what has emerged seems very different from what was envisaged. One can step back and see the brushstrokes melt away and a scheme emerge whose organization was never planned or expected. It is suddenly clear that the transformation of experiences into a book has changed oneself; in becoming part of one's history it alters the person who views what has gone on as well as altering his view of the world outside.

For instance, I find on looking inward that a rather particular admiration and fondness has grown up in my feelings for these children which I think can be separated off from feelings towards the analytic work or method, the friends involved, the great amount of the time-of-my-life expended, etc. No, it is a special admiration for these children and, in a way, for autism. I can see that, for instance, in the text I have made links to Oates, Lincoln, the fable of the True Cross, Crusaders. Clearly I feel something heroic in these children and see, albeit exaggerated and incapacitating, the germ of some greatness, some 'leap into the dark', as Kierkegaard would call it. I suspect that I am witnessing his 'knight of faith' gone wrong at the start, the eccentricity of the true individual hypertrophied beyond its root-system in psychic reality. It is my impression that this countertransference of mine is shared by those who actually worked with and knew the children. I only actually met one of them, Barry, and that was in consultation before his analysis. My own countertransference is to the group as a compound individual whose history is arranged as are the Chapters 3 to 6. It is this vertex that I wish to explore as a way of drawing together the material of the volume.

Let us start with a theoretical problem and then return to the children. There have been only two compelling addenda to Freud's conception of mental life's commencement in the baby, namely his idea of primary narcissism as a state in which identification with satisfying objects was immediate, automatic. These amplifications were first Melanie Klein's description of the primal splitting-and-idealization of self and object, originally the breast (meaning the mother as breast). By this operation the child laid the foundations for concepts of good and bad, albeit grossly exaggerated and immediate in criteria. This was considered by Melanie Klein to mark the commencement of object relations conducive to healthy development, a *sine qua non*. The second corollary was added by Esther Bick in 1968 with her description of the psychic function of the skin in mental development. She convincingly demonstrated the need for an experience of a containing object with which the baby can be identified in order to feel sufficiently contained within its own skin to be able to bear being put down by the mother in a waking state without disintegration of the body-self. She traced some of the consequences for ego-strength of a defective psychic skin and showed how substitute, second-skin functions are established to bolster the defect. Bick saw this as a prerequisite to adequate splitting and-idealization, and therefore to the satisfactory resolution of good–bad confusions.

The massive material of the clinical chapters of this book declares unequivocally that we are dealing with children in whom both these steps in development were either lost or inadequate to begin with. But we do not find the usual proliferation of persecutory anxieties, paranoid suspicions and sadistic perversity. On the contrary, the children are gentle, tender, easily cast into despairing depression, more irritated than frightened by their omnipresent rival-babies. It is only after the analysis and development has proceeded a certain distance that narcissistic hardness and cruelty with consequent persecutory fears and paranoid suspicion makes its appearance in Timmy or John. Even Barry is very little frightened of persecutors but rather is persecuted by the depressive feelings engendered by his continual damage to his object from brutal intrusiveness (the holiday bandaging for instance) and did not develop a narcissistic organization until after the establishment of an internal world and the splitting-and-idealization of self and objects ('now I know why I am ugly'). The second five years of his analysis, the last year with Timmy and with John, were all taken up with the analysis of the narcissistic organization (the John-and-Teddy head-banging manic team, for instance). Piffie, on the other hand, began his analysis with Mrs Hoxter in a state that Barry was barely to reach after nine years. It is in this sense that the children are strung together as a compound individual in my mind, illustrating the outward changes in the balance of love and hate that would ordinarily appear as matters of temperament but can be seen here to be consequences of change in personality structure. On the road to improved structure the children became more manifestly cruel and hard as splitting-and-idealization made narcissistic organization possible.

Now there is some sort of lesson hidden in these findings, something having to do with splitting-and-idealization, of good and evil as mental categories, something that raises a question about their necessity. The charge that Milton made Satan the hero of Paradise Lost is perhaps not without substance, for not many men can be seen to have struggled as Milton did to contain and deal personally, responsibly, with every aspect of himself vis à vis his object, God. It is clear that Melanie Klein viewed splitting processes as being instituted violently, by destructive impulses, regardless of the purpose or motive behind their deployment. The consequence of splitting was seen by her as always damaging to the object to some degree and therefore an occasion of guilt and remorse. And it is true, as we study splitting processes, they do have the quality of a judgment handed down and executed, regardless of the wisdom of Solomon that may lie behind it. There is an 'irritable reaching after fact and reason', a quest for the 'final solution' to the X-ish problem.

But it is also perhaps true that splitting processes are necessary for the kind of decisions that make action in the outside world possible. Every decision involves the setting in motion of a single plan from amongst its alternatives; it is experimental, involves risk, a certain ruthlessness toward oneself or others. I remember as a schoolboy being shown a science film on crystallography dealing with the cutting of a huge rough diamond of very great value. The cutters studied its structure, drew lines of its presumptive natural cleavages, and then, at the moment of great suspense, applied a little chisel, gave it a tiny tap, and the diamond fell into two clean parts. I was greatly impressed. But I am also greatly impressed by the fourteen-year-old Piffie's dream of a precious object that has natural lines of cleavage. While Mrs Bick may have discovered the secret of ego-strength, Piffie has perhaps discovered the secret of ego-resilience, of stooping-to-conquer, the reeds that bend while the oak goes down before the gale. In a word, temporizing by disengagement. Lincoln's order to his recruits would be the case in point.

Temporizing immediately raises the spectre of hesitation, indecision, procrastination, compromise, hallmark of the obsessional character. Where does the difference lie? In what way is Piffie's obsessionality different from that of Freud's Rat Man? One clear answer is that Freud's patient deployed his obsessional separating and controlling in the interest of his ambivalence to his 'lady', his love and hate. Piffie's obsessionality does not serve his ambivalence, which is in fact very little in evidence. Truly his omnipotent control is meant to subserve his desire to possess his Mrs Hoxter just as completely as John wants his 'lady', but through understanding of her inner workings, not force, ultimately. Like Barry's Mr McGoo, Piffie is a lover and wishes to understand his object so well that he can make it so blissful that it will not need, or want, other babies or daddy-penises. A primitive form of love? Yes. Egocentric? Yes. But authentic!

I must also pause at this moment to pay heed to a phenomenon not infrequent in my scientific wanderings on the ice-cap.

Whenever I approach a new landmark, I find on it a small cache of rocks and a little flag with the letter 'B', for Bion, presumably. You will have noted that we have come round to the vertices L, H, and K; love, hate and knowledge. In Bionese I seem to be suggesting that the difference between Piffie and the Rat-Man is one of vertices to their obsessionality, L and H for the Rat-Man, K for Piffie. Thus we find that the lover, the artist and the scientist are the same person and that science can start very early. But it can also outgrow its source and proliferate as an illness. This would also imply the possibility of its not doing so, and of a type of healthy, resilient personality structure being erected by means not involving splitting-and-idealization. From this viewpoint the concepts of good and evil would not be necessary in the way described by Money-Kyrle in his investigation of the internal logic of development of the mind. I would also point out that this inquiry takes us back to Melanie Klein's early emphasis on the epistemophilic instinct as a driving force in development and the mother's body as the original 'world' it explored.

This opens a window on the psychoanalytical method as a thing-in-itself that people can participate in, sometimes as the patient, sometimes as the analyst, eventually as both simultaneously. What is the emotionality stirred by this sort of experience? If the process is one dominated by Vertex of K, its essential events will be ones of becoming both knowing and known, something perhaps more Quixotic than Freud's self appellation of 'conquistador'. But essentially the process would seem to deserve the name 'adventure' and, at moments of fruition, would seem most appropriately accompanied – no, not accompanied, suffused – suffused with the feeling of wonder at the beauty of the world of the mind, the only world we can really 'know'.

Barry seems to have had his trip to the moon, and his sleep in the coffin from which he was rescued by a 'friend'. When he looked up, which Miss Weddell suggests means that he looked up at the mother's nipple instead of down at her bottom – when he looked up everything was changed. He was filled with wonder at an object that could rescue him in his sleep, without his giving it the slightest assistance, by talking its psychoanalytical music of PATV, DWTV, and PAC – the psychoanalytic conspiracy. His distrust of PAC centred on his suspicion that its ultimate goal was to get him away from his mother to enable him to earn a living. There was probably more than a grain of truth in this, though it should not have been so. Psychoanalysts should, of course, have no goal but that of carrying on analytic processes. But that is part of the difficulty of K and its field of uncertainty; it forbids us to have goals and external criteria, and this places us in a position very vulnerable indeed to criticism and ridicule.

It is precisely in relation to such difficulties that the distinction between strength and resilience appears. Milton's Samson was strong in his belief in God before he fell to Dalila's seduction. But eyeless in Gaza he was resilient, could resist seduction, temporize with threats and await his opportunity:

Commands are not constraints. If I obey them,
I do it freely, venturing to displease
God for the fear of man, and man prefer,
Set God behind: (*Samson Agonistes*, ll. 1375–1378)
. . .
Master's commands come with a power resistless
To such as owe them absolute subjection;
And for a life who will not change his purpose?
(So mutable are the ways of men).
Yet this be sure, in nothing to comply
Scandalous or forbidden in our law.   (1409–1414).

The essential difference lies in the shift from the splitting-and-idealization which equates the nation of Israel with God and good, while the Philistines and Dagon are evil, to the differentiation between the internal world of God and Law and the external world of friends and enemies; yesterday's friends being today's enemies and perhaps tomorrow's friends once more. Whereas good and evil are created by violent splitting and idealization, the differentiation internal–external follows a line of cleavage, needs only a little tap on the chisel, can be painlessly put together again, like Piffie's beautiful shelter.

Abraham, K. (1945). *Selected Papers*. London: Hogarth.

Bick, E. (1968). The experience of the skin in early object relations. *International Journal of Psychoanalysis*, 49: 484–486.

Bion, W. R. (1962). Learning from Experience. London: Heinemann.

Bion, W.R.(1963). *The Elements of Psychoanalysis*. London: Heinemann.

Bion, W. R. (1965). *Transformations*. London: Heinemann.

Bion, W. R. (1967). *Second Thoughts*. London: Heinemann.

Bion, W. R. (1970). *Attention and Interpretation*. London: Tavistock.

Cassirer, E. (1955). *The Philosophy of Symbolic Forms*. Oxford: O.U.P.

Chomsky, N. (1966). *Cartesian Linguistics*. New York: Harper.

Chomsky, N. (1968). *Syntactic Structures*. The Hague: Mouton.

Freud, S. (1893). *Studies on Hysteria* (with J. Breuer). *S. E.*, II

Freud, S. (1900). *The Interpretation of Dreams. S. E.*, IV and V.

Freud, S. (1905). Fragment of a case of hysteria [Dora]. *S. E.*, VII.

Freud, S. (1905). *Three Essays on Sexuality. S. E.*, VII.

Freud, S. (1909). Analysis of a phobia in a five-year-old boy [Little Hans]. *S. E.*, X.

Freud, S. (1909). Notes upon a case of obsessional neurosis ['Rat Man']. *S. E.*, X.

Freud, S. (1910). Leonardo da Vinci and a memory of his childhood. *S.E.*, XI.

Freud, S. (1911). Notes on an autobiographical account of a case of paranoia [Schreber case]. *S. E.*, XI.

Freud, S. (1914). On narcissism: an introduction. *S. E.*, XIV.

Freud, S. (1915). Repression. *S. E.*, XIV.

Freud, S. (1917). *Mourning and Melancholia. S. E.*, XIV.

Freud, S. (1918). From the history of an infantile neurosis ['Wolf Man']. *S. E.*, XVII.

Freud, S. (1919). A child is being beaten. *S. E.*, XVII.

Freud, S. (1923). The ego and the id. *S. E.*, XIX.

Freud, S. (1938). Splitting of the ego in the process of defence. *S. E.*, XXII.

Geach, P. (1957). Mental Acts. London: Routledge.

Klein, M. (1932). *The Psychoanalysis of Children.* London: Hogarth.

Klein, M. (1948). *Contributions to Psychoanalysis* (1921–1945). London: Hogarth.

Klein, M. (1952). *Developments in Psychoanalysis* (with P. Heimann, S. Isaacs and J. Riviere). London: Hogarth.

Klein, M. (1957). *Envy and Gratitude.* London: Tavistock.

Klein, M. (1961). *Narrative of a Child Analysis* [Richard]. London: Hogarth.

Jakobson, R. and Halle, M. (1955). *Fundamentals of Language.* The Hague: Mouton.

Langer, S. K. (1942). *Philosophy in a New Key.* New York: Harper.

Meltzer, D. (1967). *The Psychoanalytical Process.* London: Heinemann.

Meltzer, D. (1973). *Sexual States of Mind.* Strathtay: Clunie Press.

Money-Kyrle, R. (1961). *Man's Picture of His World.* London: Duckworth.

Russell, B. (1940). *An Inquiry into Meaning and Truth.* London: Allen & Unwin.

Sandberg, C. (1926). *Abraham Lincoln – The Prairie Years.* New York: Harcourt, Brace.

Tustin, F. (1972). *Autism and Childhood Psychosis.* London: Hogarth.

Whitehead, A. N. (1933). *Adventures in Ideas.* Cambridge: C.U.P.

Winnicott, D. W. (1957). *Collected Papers: Through Paediatrics to Psychoanalysis.* London: Tavistock.

Wittgenstein, L. (1945). *Philosophical Investigations.* Oxford: Blackwell.

List of patients and analysts

Baby Alice (Mrs Bick) 230
Barry (Doreen Weddell) 6, 15, 26, 27, 32, 97–156, 224, 227
Jill (Mrs Bick) 232
John (Isca Wittenberg) 9, 14, 19, 55–96, 227, 239
Jonathan (Donald Meltzer) 191
Mary (Mrs Bick) 231
neurotic man (Mrs Bick) 232
Phillipa (Donald Meltzer) 194
Piffie (Shirley Hoxter) 15, 23, 25, 157–188, 206–214
schizoid girl (Donald Meltzer) 214–216
Sylvia (Donald Meltzer) 191–193
Timmy (John Bremner) 6, 8, 14, 19, 20, 33–53

Chronology of treatment processes

Timmy (autism proper)
history 33
autism proper (15th session) 37

sensual relation to objects 37
dismantling of senses 38, 47
two-dimensional relation to space 39
geographical confusion 38
clearing of transference space-time 40
       cordonning 40
       mirror behaviour 40
       under-the-analyst's chair 41
       analyst's head-breast 41
introjection and projection 41
       'squeezing' material 41
       delusional jealousy 39
       intolerance of separation 41
       projective identification 42
       language development 43
therapeutic achievement 44
reconstruction 45

John (primal depression)

history 58
invasiveness ('the meteor') 57
suicidal impulse ('the tip-up lorry') 59
inside-outside confusion 60
splitting-and-idealization ('thrown away') 60
reversible perspective 60
regression 62
integration of combined part-object 63, 68
despair 69, 79
oedipal triumph 76
passivity of object 65
sparing of object 65
language development ('the Laby') 66
adhesive identification 66, 82
differentiation of boundaries ('Lady gone') 69
increased physical vulnerability 69
relation to time 70
manic expulsion 72, 75
narcissistic organization (with Teddy) 69
reality-testing impairment 70

top–bottom differentiation 71
fear of loss (getting-in–keeping-out') 71
combined object 72, 76, 77, 79, 96
restitution 72
erotization of nipple 73
depression ('insider or outsider') 77, 87
reintrojection of expelled object ('intrusion and collapse')
    74
attractiveness of breast ('roses, roses') 76
perverse trends ('at the taps') 78
projection of depression ('all mine') 79, 85
possessiveness of inside of breast ('abandoned to
    mindlessness') 84
narcissistic organization as defence against depression 85
negativism 89
attacks on linking 90
fetishistic object 89

Barry (disturbed geography)

history 99
eyes as vehicle of oral sadism and invasiveness 103
reversible perspective 103
identification with damaged objects 104
passivity of object (effigy dream) 105
intolerance of separation (handing-over technique) 105
manic reparation 107
paper-thin object 108
policeman-penis (*drawings* i–viii) 109
breast–bottom–baby confusion 117
internal–external differentiation (*drawings* ix–xiv) 121
compartmentalization of internal space 117, 125
intrusive *versus* helpful projective identification 126
fear of death-of-the-breast (*drawing* xv) 127
zonal confusion (*drawing* xvi) 131
authority of the combined object 135, 149
lessened omnipotence (*drawing* xvii) 137
memory function 139
technical handling of violence 141

attacks on primal scene (*drawing* xviii) 143
relation of internal to external anxieties 145
attacks on meaning of words (*drawing* xix) 148
improved containment 151
introjective identification with combined part-object
      151
  dreams: coffin 151
      landing on the moon 151
      emperor of the moon 151
      family train 154
confusion of bad and damaged objects 155

Piffie (residual autism)

history 158
obsessive orderliness 160
container-lap 160
    and language development 161
    and fragments of self 162
deceptive progress 162
segmenting and assembling 162–163
    compared with splitting-and-idealization 163
intrusion into object 164–165
    man-on-the-ladder episode 165
manic reparation 165
    Piffie-the-plumber 165, 172
reparation 165
    torn-drawing material 166
obsessive incorporation 166
    'carpets' 167
    relation to memory 167
    'parcels', cat-shop material 168
stylized and bizarre movements, origin of 169
    and exchange of identity 172
interruption of treatment 172
    comparison with Timmy 171
relation to nipple 172
    as nipple-penis 172
    linking 172

relation to time 172
second period of treatment 173
baby–schoolboy split 174
obsessionality 174
 records 174, 176
 control of language 176
 research interests 177
 litigiousness (Mrs Hoxter's-lateness episode) 178
 sophisticated employment ('crazy-paving' dream) 179
 control of primal scene ('Chi-Chi the panda' dream) 181
 diminution ('King of Nepal' dream) 181
 comparison with Barry 183
 creative employment ('beautiful shelter' dream) 185

Abraham, K. 219
adhesive identification 68, 94,
    204–206, 230–240
    vs. projective identification
    229
attention, nature of 11–12, 14
    containing quality 98, 234
    and dismantling 15, 23, 205
    in post-autism 26
auditory containment, in autism
    19
autism proper 5, 8–15, 35–56
    dynamic aspects 12
    economic factors 8
    genetic considerations 15
    and personality development
    15
    prerequisite mental traits 8–15
    organization of life-space 17
    organization of self and objects
    22
    structural characteristics 10

Bick, E.
    and adhesive identification
    92, 204, 230
    and Bion's container–con-
    tained 48, 58, 154, 157,
    240
    differentiation of inadequate
    container in autism 19, 237
    integrity of object 99, 106,109
    'The experience of the skin in
    early object relations 233–236,
    242
Bion, W. R.
    absent breast/object 95, 215,
    227
    alpha-function 23, 201, 215,
    217
    attacks on linking 92
    'common sense' 12, 91, 203,
    217
    container–contained 46, 154,
    189, 240

L, H, K (vertices) 245
maternal reverie 22, 58, 99,
    157, 158, 192
nameless dread 154
reverse perspective 62, 156
breast, as object 15, 83, 110, 119,
    155, 242
    absent 95
    confusion around 121, 130
    containing function 98, 129,
        152, 188
    head-breast of analyst 46, 53,
        84, 143
    hope-breast 65, 72
    paper-thin 22
    scattered sensorily 53
    separation from nipple 211
    toilet-breast 84, 152, 157,
        213
    see also combined object
Cassirer, E. 217
Chomsky, N. 192, 201
combined object 65, 78, 83, 120,
    137, 154, 155
common sense (consensuality) 12,
    18, 23, 40, 91, 203, 217
compartmentalization of internal
    space 40, 119, 161, 166, 178,
    185, 226
confusion
    baby-in-breast 121
    geographical 17–18, 41, 60
    zonal 133
containment
    failure of 19, 54, 235
    and language development
        19, 45, 134, 154, 164, 168,
        191–206
    and three-dimensional object
        96, 233
deafness (apparent) 19, 25, 101,
    160, 188

death-of-the-breast, fear of 129,
    152, 176, 188
denial of psychic reality vs. two-
    dimensionality 240
depressive collapse 19, 47, 57, 74,
    92
diagnosis, problems of 33
dimensionality 225–240
    impairment of 28
    'life-space' or 'geography of
        phantasy' 12, 17, 27, 41,
        64, 127, 223
    'life-time' 15, 226
    one-dimensionality 226
    paper-thin object 22
    two-dimensionality 18, 22,
        41, 51, 97, 227
    three-dimensionality 96, 228
    four-dimensionality 225
disintegration 164, 188, 203, 242
    vs. unintegration 234
dismantling 3, 10, 11–12, 23–29,
    40, 165, 173, 203, 217,
    220
    distinction from splitting 11,
        164
    Piffie's dream 187
    and transitional objects/fetish
        27, 48
Ferenczi, S. 230
fetishism, relation to dismantling
    25, 27, 28, 49, 91
forgetfulness
    vs. repression 218
    see also memory
Freud, S.
    'choice of neurosis' 209
    linearity of theory 226
    mental functions vs. mental
        events 240
    on obsessionality 244
    'organ' of consciousness 12

on personality structure 16, 227, 229
primary narcissism 21
on repetition compulsion 13
on repression 218
on splitting 23
on thought 20
Geach, P. 215–217
geography of phantasy 17, 128, 151, 206, 226
   ee also dimensionality
internal space 19, 47, 67, 96, 116, 127, 1340 142, 172, 174, 204, 227, 233
   see also geography of phantasy
introjective processes 45, 54, 78, 99, 154, 156, 204, 230, 233
   concrete 169, 174
   vs. dismantling 24, 227
   and projective 93, 141, 230
   and separateness of object 94, 158, 188
   of speaking object 193, 200, 201
Jakobson, R. 192
Kierkegaard, S. 199, 242
Klein, M.
   on breast as object 158
   on epistemophilic drive 166, 220, 245
   method of child analysis 1, 2
   on splitting processes 23–24, 226, 230, 242, 243
Langer, S. 191, 217
language development 19, 44, 134, 146, 164, 168, 191–206
   see also mutism; symbol formation
Levin, K. 225

linking, attacks on 11, 22, 23, 54, 92
   nipple as model 174
manic/omnipotent reparation 98, 111, 167, 211
Melville, H. 27
memory 52, 67, 96, 141, 169, 186, 199, 201, 218, 227
   see also forgetfulness
mental acts 12, 217
Merleau Ponti, M. 192
Milton, J. 243, 246
mindlessness
   abandonment to 86
   in autism proper 10, 14, 32, 36, 203, 227
   and countertransference 173
   vs. developmental process 45
   in everyday life 3
   and mutism 204
   and shallowness 237
   as temporizing move 3, 244
Money-Kyrle, R. 155, 245
mutism 19, 31, 41, 191–206, 217
   see also language development
narcissistic identification 229
   adhesive 204
   and dimensionality 225
   primary, and post-autistic 21, 242
   and speaking object 192
   and transitional object 27
   vs. quest for good object 221, 229
nipple, as part-object 66, 74, 79, 80, 83, 85, 90, 116, 143, 154
   organizing function 94, 97, 174
   see also combined object
object *see* breast; combined object; dimensionality

obsessionality 21–28, 178–187
    balance/modulation 221
    creative use of 219, 222
    dismantling/segmenting 165
    L, H, K vertices 245
    primitive mechanisms
        168–172
    'scientific' (Piffie) 210
play disruption *vs.* autistic disruption 6
possessiveness 19, 50, 66, 93, 106
post-autistic personality 9, 16,
        19–22, 25–29, 215, 231,
        237
    similar to newborn 21
primal scene 145, 183
    see also combined object
projective identification 60, 93,
        141, 154, 197, 230
    as communication 192
    and concept of internal space
        204
    with dead objects 157
    intrusive vs. helpful 99, 128,
        156
    vs. symbolic form 217
reparation see manic reparation
repetition compulsion 13
Russell, B. 191, 217
'second-skin' formation 234, 237,
    242
shallowness of character 237–240

splitting
    diamond-cutting analogy 244
    vs. dismantling 11, 48, 164,
        203
    Freud on 240
    and idealization 9, 141, 226,
        237, 242, 246
    Klein's paper 24, 233
symbol formation 217, 218
    impaired 20,51, 52, 172
    symbolic equation 170
    see also language development; mutism
technique 14, 40, 92, 142
time, attitudes to 7, 9, 10, 13, 39,
        70, 155, 158, 172, 180,
        199, 226–229, 237
    in autism proper 15, 28
    in catatonia 218
    see also dimensionality
transference, as core method of
        investigation 2, 6, 7, 14,
        33–36, 193, 199, 209, 220
    and countertransference 101,
        104, 119, 128, 140, 173,
        242
transitional object 18, 27, 28
Tustin, F. 94, 204
Whitehead, A. N. 7
Winnicott, D. W. 18, 27
Wittgenstein, L. 191, 192, 202,
    203